The Magic of Rice

Knowing more about Rice

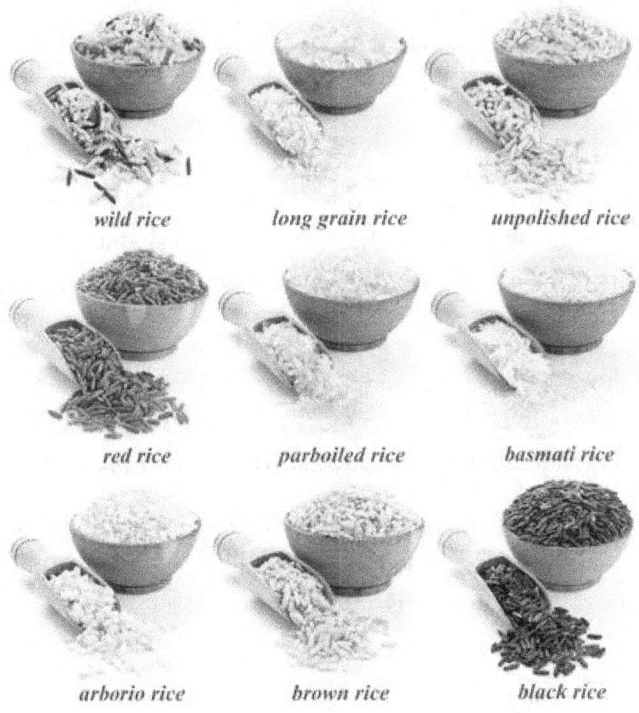

wild rice   long grain rice   unpolished rice

red rice   parboiled rice   basmati rice

arborio rice   brown rice   black rice

Health Learning Series

Dueep Jyot Singh

Mendon Cottage Books

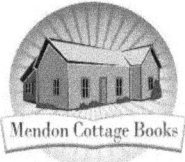

Mendon Cottage Books

JD-Biz Publishing

Disclaimer

The information is this book is provided for informational purposes only. It is not intended to be used and medical advice or a substitute for proper medical treatment by a qualified health care provider. The information is believed to be accurate as presented based on research by the author.

The contents have not been evaluated by the U.S. Food and Drug Administration or any other Government or Health Organization and the contents in this book are not to be used to treat cure or prevent disease.

The author or publisher is not responsible for the use or safety of any diet, procedure or treatment mentioned in this book. The author or publisher is not responsible for errors or omissions that may exist.

Warning

The Book is for informational purposes only and before taking on any diet, treatment or medical procedure, it is recommended to consult with your primary health care provider.

Our books are available at

1. Amazon.com
2. Barnes and Noble
3. Itunes
4. Kobo
5. Smashwords
6. Google Play Books

Table of Contents

The Magic of Rice...1

    Introduction..4
    Growing Rice in Your Garden 8
    Harvesting Your Rice...13
    Types of Rice 17
        Difference between Parboiled Rice and Instant Rice.........................18

    Pests and Diseases..19
        Pesticides and Botanicals 20

    Popular Rice Cultivars 22
    Rice Dishes 23
        Cooking Rice..25

        Reviving Overcooked Rice 31

        Steamed Rice..32

    Traditional Pilavs and Biriyanis..33
        Savory Pilau With Chicken..33

        Biryani...35

        Traditional Biryani – spiced Meat Pilau 36

    Brown Rice and Polished Rice..40
    Conclusion 44
    Author Bio...47
    Publisher...58

Introduction

Bless that hungry nomad millenniums ago, who while traveling over the grasslands, suddenly found that there was a wild grass growing and its seed when collected could be cooked and eaten to provide him and his hungry family with the most nourishing food available.

This is an ordinary grain of rice, a grass growing all over the world, and consumed thankfully by millions globally, every day. In fact, it is the staple diet of the major population in Asia. "Rice bowls" of the world are places where rice is grown extensively and which feed not only the native population, but the population of other parts of the world.

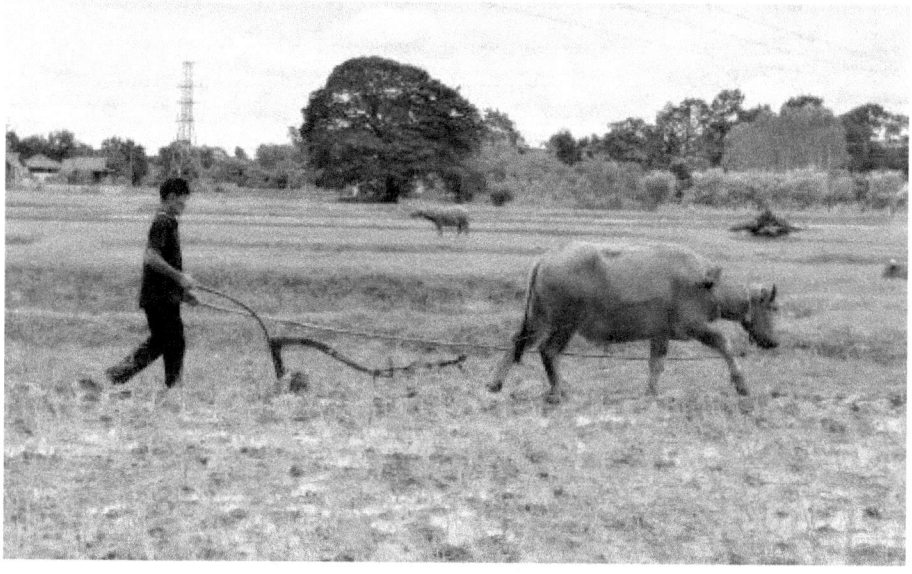

Old ancient traditional ways of cultivating rice are still being followed in many parts of the world today, especially in Asia.

1/5 of all the calories that you are eating in your meals may be the gift of rice, if you are a native of Asia or other Eastern countries. According to historical legend and excavations, rice was first domesticated in the Chinese region more than 15,000 years ago! From here, it spread all over South Asia and Southeast Asia. Human migrations as well as trading routes opening up as time went by spread rice globally, and to the west.

Thanks to European colonization and trading, rice began to be grown in other parts of the world, and even though it did not have such a sacred part in the traditional, social and time-honored customs of the East, its value as a nourishing cereal was accepted globally as time went by.

People in other parts of the globe, especially in Italy and Spain soon found out that this grain could be grown profitably in their own lands. That was because the climate was ideal and suitable for rice growing. On the other hand, rice cannot be grown in England, because of the cold weather.

The social significance of rice goes back more than 3000 years, especially in the East, where traditional rice ceremonies were held every year, in praise of the rice goddess Dewi Sri in Java and Bali. In Indonesia and Japan, they have their own ancient rice God who is going to bless their harvest with a plentiful crop after he has been appeased in the traditional rice festival.

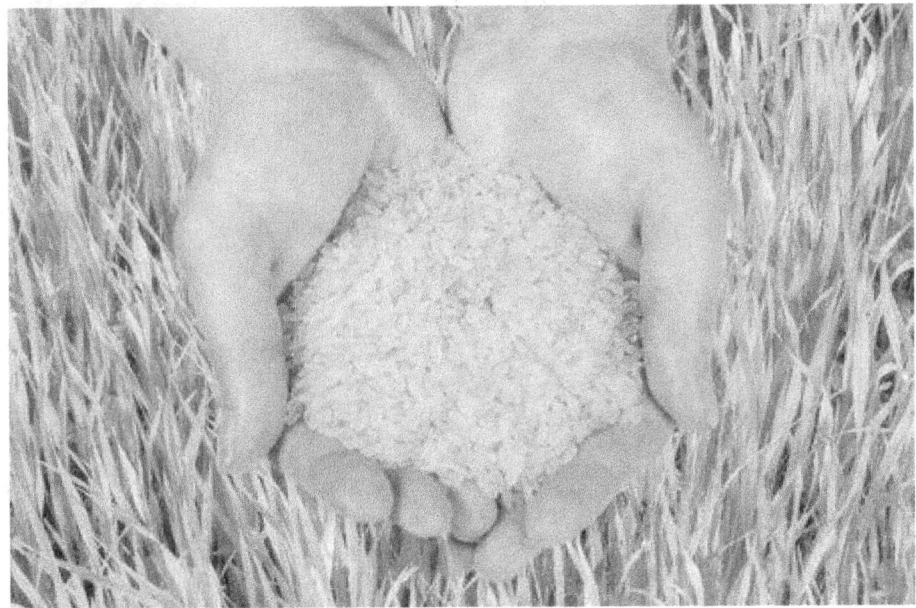

Even today, plenty of rituals in the East will never be complete without some grains of rice being offered to the gods. They may also be presented with rice wine.

Even today, in many parts of the world, a single grain of rice is considered to be holy. I remember as a child seeing a neighbor feeding her hungry brood and admonishing them to clear up their plates. Not a single grain of rice was left.

I, not being a born rice eater, was rather surprised at this stricture, and thought a bit of typical bossy adult fuss. But that lady, who was very highly educated and cultured, told me that their native tradition demanded they always ate the last grain of rice on the plate with eyes closed and thanking God for the meal.

That last grain was a gift To Him, and Which Would Feed Him!

I was of course very impressed with this tradition, and even though I as a rather cynical adult would listen to it without being overly impressed, I think it is an excellent way to get children to finish up everything on their plates without fussing!

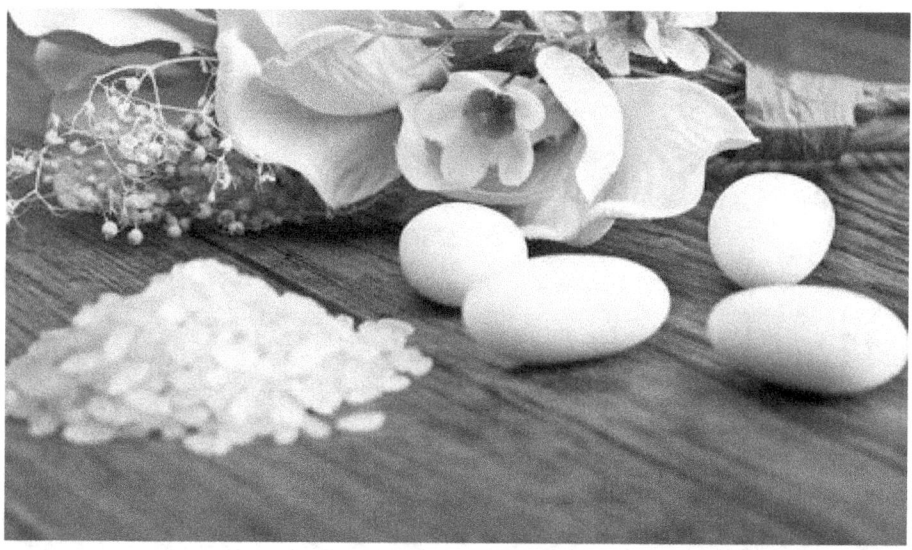

Rice, confetti and flowers during the wedding are all very nice, but eggs?

In many ancient Asian cultures, the rice goddess made a link between Earth and Heaven, with rice. The pagan tradition of throwing rice on the newlywed bride and groom goes back to millenniums. This is done even in Christian weddings, without people thinking about its significance. The origin is pagan, asking the blessings of the old gods to bless the newlywed couple with plenty of food in the shape of rice, and also many children.[1]

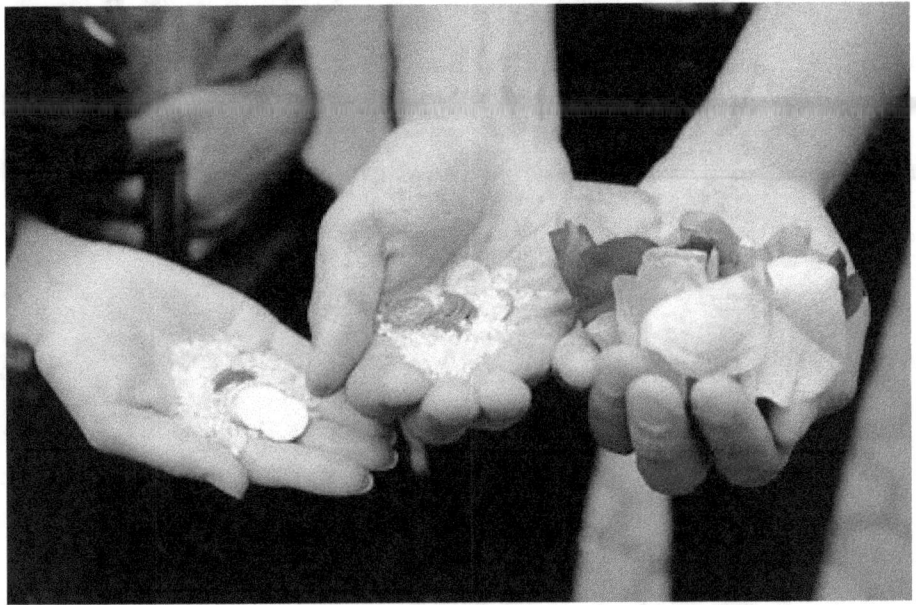

Getting ready for the arrival of the newlywed bride and groom.

---

[1] Almost as many children as there were grains of rice thrown on the couple! But that was the time when more children meant more chances of the tribe surviving from the depredations of their enemies and disease.

You may like to hear more about rice in weddings in this particular URL, with Greer Garson imitating the patter of the immortal Sir Harry Lauder – Movie Random Harvest, Song - She's Ma Daisy-

https://www.youtube.com/watch?v=rcH-tVCwhWc

Growing Rice in Your Garden

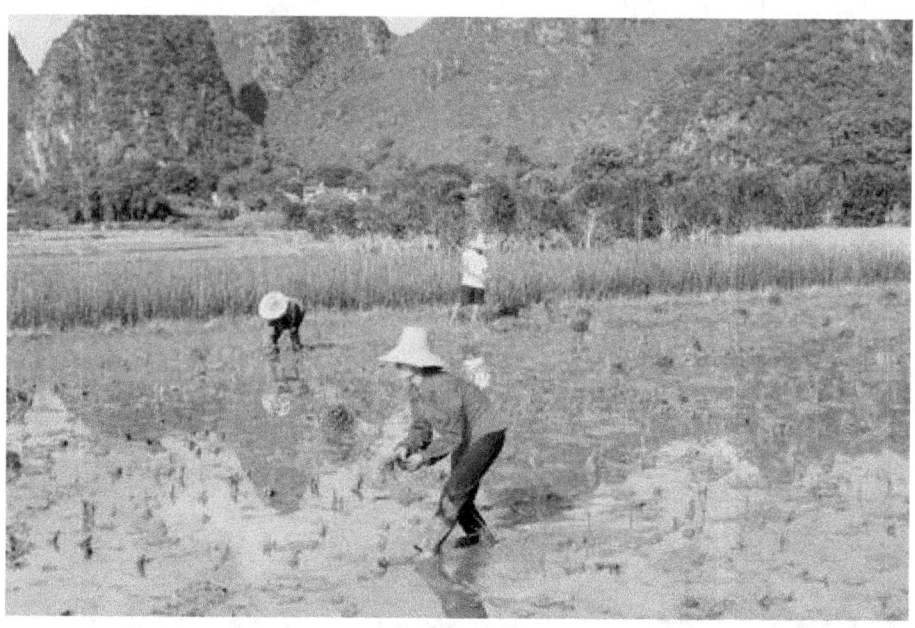

Many of us are under the impression that for growing rice, you need wide-open spaces, like in China, the Nile Delta or the plains of Missouri, Mississippi, Texas, and Arkansas where rice is being grown extensively. That is not so. You can even grow rice in your own backyard, in a container, or even on your terrace. I know about a friend, who grows rice on his porch. But he was the person who grew wheat on his terrace!

If you find yourself driving down North of Sacramento in California, you are going to see lots of rice fields. California got to know about rice, during the Gold Rush when Chinese immigrants brought rice along with them, especially the medium and the short grain variety.

Rice growing has not been very successful in Australia, even though there is plenty of sun and water there because of the high toxic levels of manganese and iron in the soil.

The best temperature for growing rice is 20°C, but the temperature should not go beyond 40°C.

There is an old saying in the East about rice. For human beings to flourish, you can have your head wet. But your feet need to be dry. But that does not work for rice. Its head should be dry, but its feet should be wet!

The secret of growing rice is that you have to create an artificial rice paddy field so that your rice can thrive. In Thailand, Burma, and in Japan, these paddy fields flooded with water in trenches, by the sides of the growing plants are still utilized for breeding catfish and crayfish! And that is because, they are always full of water. So when you are ready to harvest your rice, you are going to have the extra benefit of readily available catfish or other delicious fish like eels to prepare a spicy gravy as accompaniment to your bowl of rice.

So here you are, with all the containers you have, for growing rice. Make sure that there are no holes in the bottom of the containers. They can be plastic buckets. They can also be plastic containers in which things came packed and which you previously intended to discard. But any container, if whole is never discarded by a creative gardener. He immediately turns the container into a receptacle for growing seedlings.

These are now receptacles for growing rice.

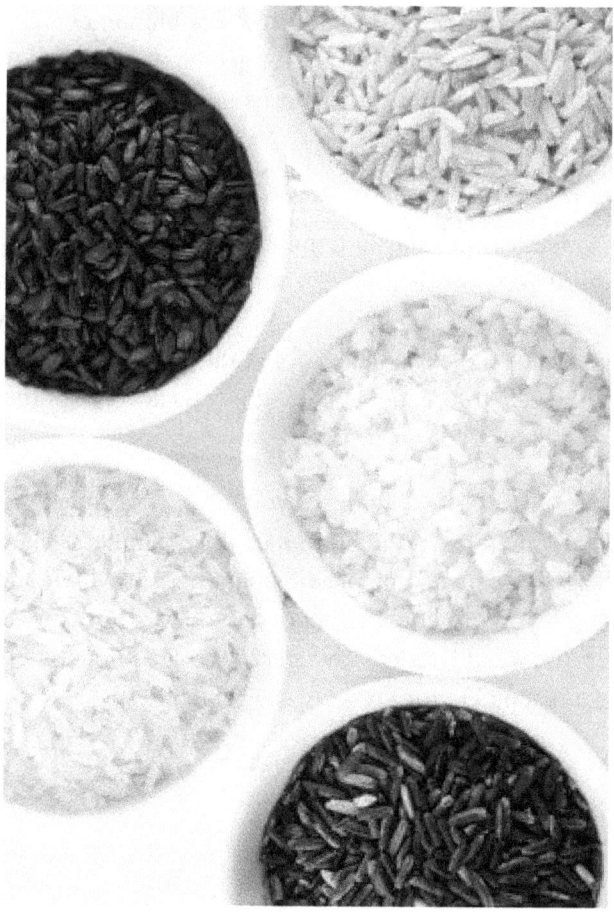

Choose the variety you want to grow from the healthy cultivars you find all over the world.

Now you have to buy the best rice seeds. I will be talking about basmati rice, later on, but those original seeds are not very easily available even to farmers in Asia. Alas, genetic engineering and carelessness has nearly wiped out the original basmati rice plant and what we have today is the sheer travesty of what our ancestors ate about hundred years ago.

Nevertheless, go to your nearest grocery store and ask for long grain wild or brown rice. If your nursery or friendly neighborhood market gardener man has already sprouted some rice grains so much the better. Organically grown rice is going to have a better chance of sprouting than rice, which has been treated before packing.

Do not buy anything which has been subjected to machine treatment or chemicals for preserving purposes. White rice does not work here, because it has already been through the processing process and it is not going to germinate, now. This rice has now been restricted to just cooking rice, thanks to the processing activity.

Rice seeds are also available in garden supply shops. Notice the seeds. They are going to be brown in color.

Fill the containers or the buckets with soil, which is rich in compost. You can also use potting compost with plenty of dirt. 6 inches is enough, because that is the amount of soil, which the rice needs in which to take root.

Now drown that soil with about 2 inches of water. After that, toss some rice seeds over the surface of the water. As the water gets absorbed in the soil, the seeds are going to sink into the wet soil. They are now going to be lying on the soil surface, but under the water.

Your job is to keep the water supply in the container from drying. Rice also likes lots of sun, and lots of warmth. That is why you need to keep all your rice containers in the sun. Make sure that they are not subject or exposed to the direct sun in the afternoons, even though they do not seem to take any harm from the direct burning heat of the sun in Asian countries.

But I would suggest less of direct sun during the day. The water level is going to be kept at a height of 2 inches, until you see your rice plants sprouting out. Once they have taken hold of the soil, you come to keeping their "feet wet. "

The plants are now about 6 inches high. The water level is now going to be increased to a depth of 4 inches. After that, let the soil absorb the water on its own, and the evaporation through the atmosphere is also going to do its own work. So by the time you are ready to harvest your rice, your rice field is going to be almost dry and the standing water will have nearly evaporated or have been absorbed.

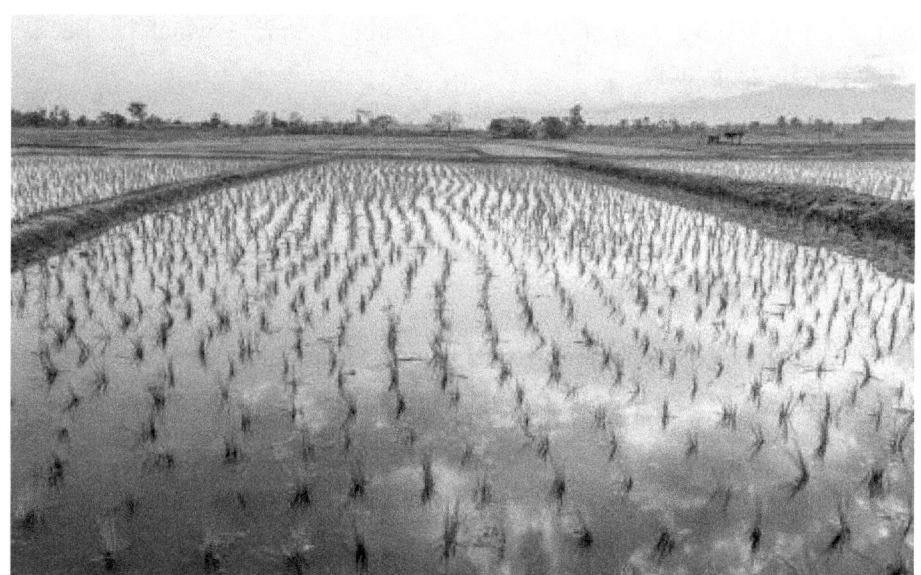

Keep their feet wet.

Harvesting Your Rice

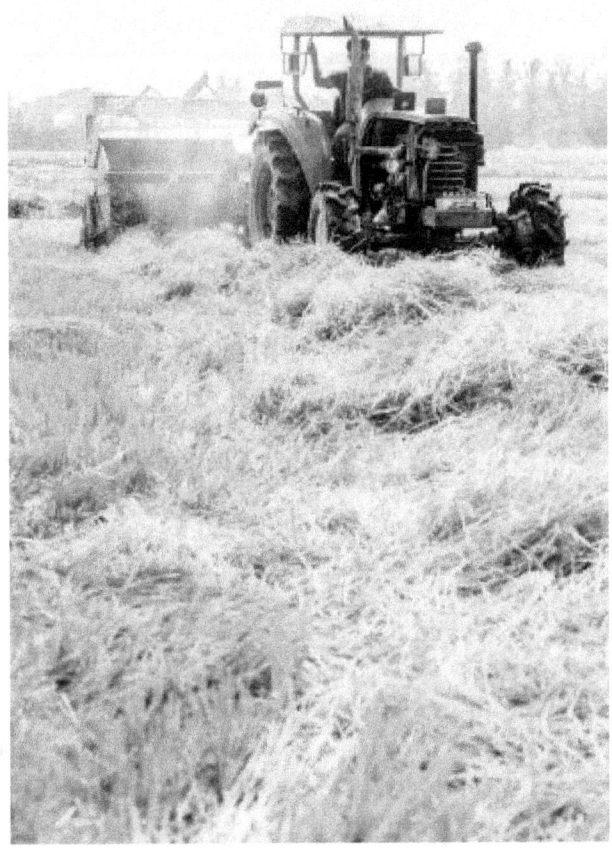

Rice is being harvested here with the help of a tractor

Rice plants mature in four months. You know that the plant is ready for harvesting because the stalk is going to change color. It is going to turn gold from green. The rice grains are now ripe. Look at them. Each grain is going to be covered with its own protective outer husk.

If there is any sort of water left in the fields, at that time, you need to drain the water out before harvesting. That is because the tops of the rice plants are going to droop and you do not want the seeds trailing in standing water, do you?

As the fields dry out completely, the grains are going to ripen even further. That is the time to harvest the panicles on which these grains have ripened.

 These panicles which are attached to the stalks are cut by harvesters in large farms, and also traditionally by hand, the old-fashioned way, with sickles and sharp knives.

These panicles are now left to dry in a dry and warm place. You can wrap them up in newspapers, to absorb the moisture, but old traditional methods advocated covering them with cotton cloths and jute sacks so that the moisture could be absorbed properly.

These panicles should also be checked regularly, during their drying period of two – three weeks to make sure that there is no sort of fungal infection brought about by moisture or water retention.

Now we come to the process of threshing. This means removing the outer husk. If I was living in a village in some remote part of the world where a rice harvest had just been garnered, I would set my cattle loose on the rice so that they could trample the husk in the process of threshing it.

After that, the rice along with the trampled husk and the seeds would be gathered in bamboo sieves and shaken vigorously, thrown up and down and swirled high up in the air in a winnowing motion. This would loosen the husks, – known as the chaff – and they would blow away in the wind, leaving the rice seeds behind. And one would sing millenniums old traditional harvesting songs in Thanksgiving at the same time.[2]

---

[2] I have been fortunate enough, to have taken part in such a threshing and de-Husking ritual when I was a child. Naturally, it left me rather covered with rather scratchy rice husks, but the singing was loud, long, enthusiastic on the part of the threshers and also very tuneless, nasal and noisy on my part. These are magic moments.

That rice gathered from the fields was later eaten with traditional fish Mouli (traditional fish curry.)

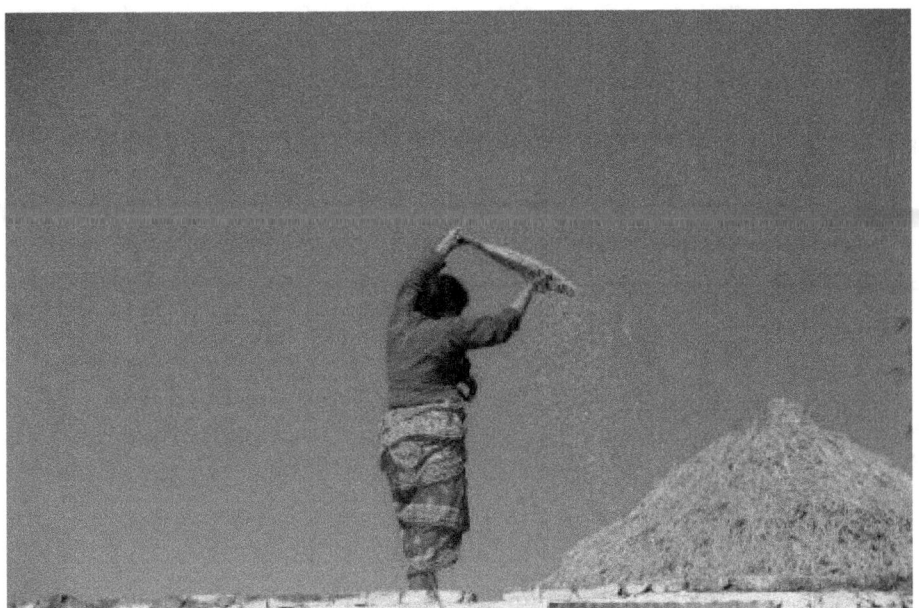

It is not as easy to do as it looks!

A rice plant depending on its variety is going to grow anywhere between 3 feet to 5 feet in height. Soil fertility is going to either reduce its height or you are going to have a 5.9 feet high rice plant.

The seeds are edible and treasured all over the world as the precious grain of rice.

For millenniums, rice has been grown extensively in areas, where the rainfall was high. It takes a lot of labor to cultivate a field of paddy, and that is why this is one of the most popular crops planted in areas where the cost of labor is negligible or low.

Paddy fields were normally flooded with water during or after the young seedlings were planted and set. This naturally needed experience, especially in the matter of channeling the water and damming it so that the seedlings do not flow away in a gush of water.

Flooding is the traditional way in which rice fields are still watered. Other methods used for irrigation purposes are going to increase the chances of pests and weeds, which keep away from flooded fields.

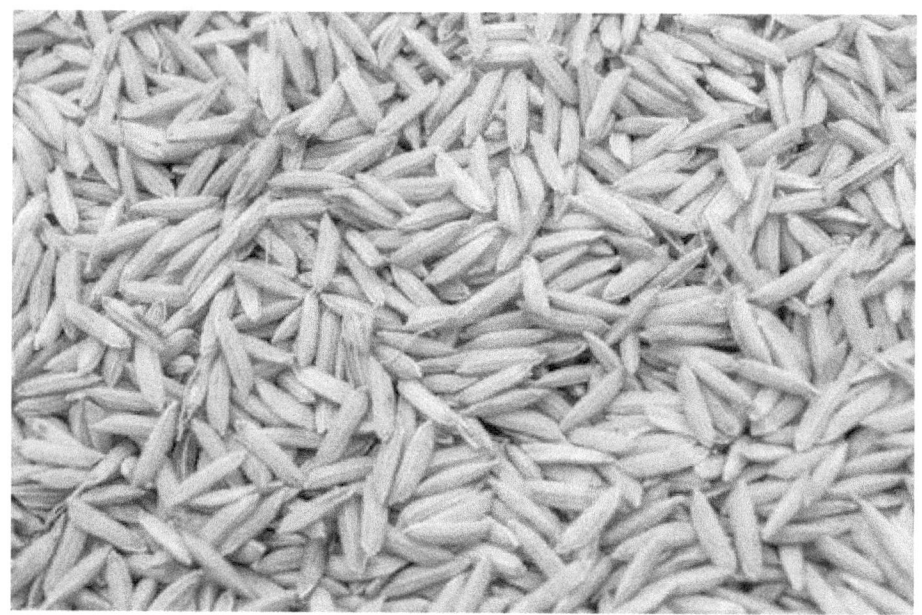

Grains of rice ready for threshing.

Types of Rice

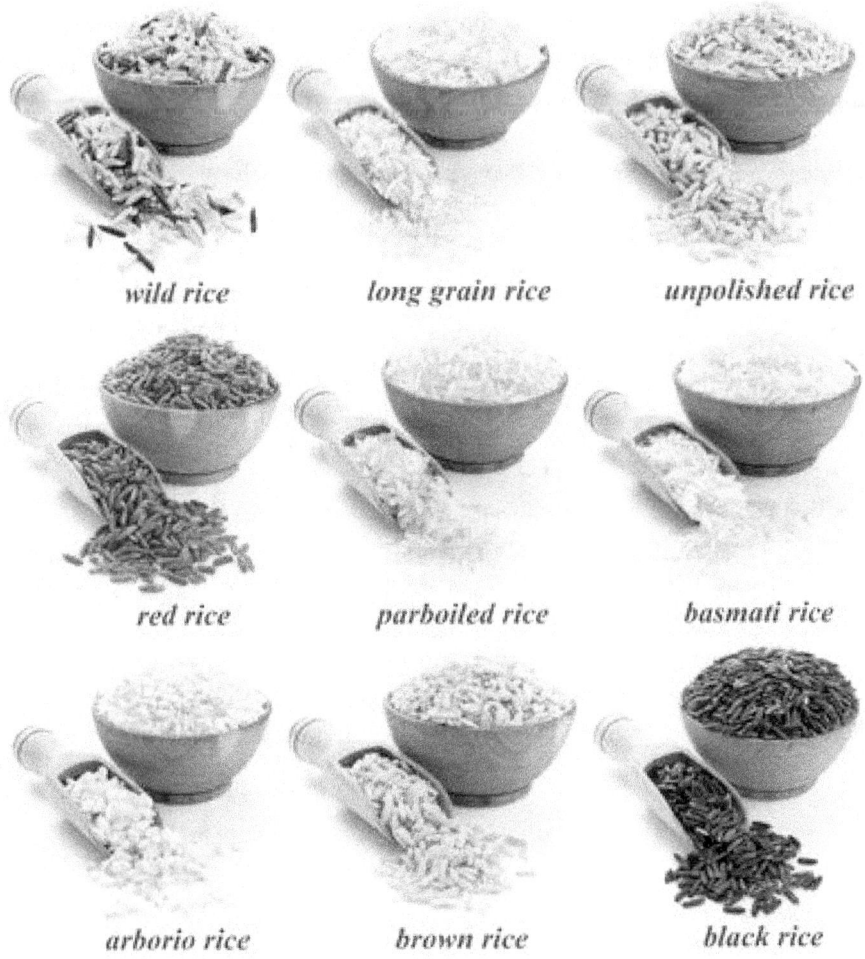

wild rice   long grain rice   unpolished rice

red rice   parboiled rice   basmati rice

arborio rice   brown rice   black rice

The different varieties of rice recognized all over the world are classified in three types, depending on the length of the grain. These are long grained, medium grained and short-grained.

Long grained rice types are held to be of greater value, because even after cooking, they are going to remain intact and separated from each other. That is why they are the best choice for rice pilavs. Medium and short grained rice are best used for boiling purposes, because even if they are clumped together, one does not feel as if he has been cheated of an aesthetically pleasing dish which is also tasty at the same time.

That is why medium grain rice is the best choice for for risotto. You can also steam rice and make them into rice dumplings as are very popular in China and in Thailand.

Sushi is made from a rice variety which can be molded, after it has been cooked. Rice pudding is best made from short grained or broken rice.

Difference between Parboiled Rice and Instant Rice

Instant Rice is cooked fully, before it is packed. All you have to do is open up the packet and microwave it, or you can microwave it in the package itself. This precooked rice is dry and dehydrated, and you are going to have a quick meal at the cost of taste, aroma, and texture.

Parboiled rice is half boiled when it is still covered with the husk. It is soaked. After that, it is subjected to steaming and drying. This parboiled rice is then processed easily by hand, because then the husk removal can be done easily.

Rice flour made from grinding rice which was left overnight is normally added to dishes and frying batter to give the food a richer texture.

Pests and Diseases

You may find your rice plants subjected to bacterial and fungal infections, because these flourish in moist and muggy atmospheres. Apart from that, soil parasites and nematodes, weeds, insects, birds and rodents are pests which are going to attack your rice crop as often as they can.

There are a number of factors that can cause a pest or disease outbreak in your rice harvest. Climactic factors include high rainfall, which is going to bring about the invasion of worms and midges. And if it is a drought season or condition, you are going to suffer from thrips.[3]

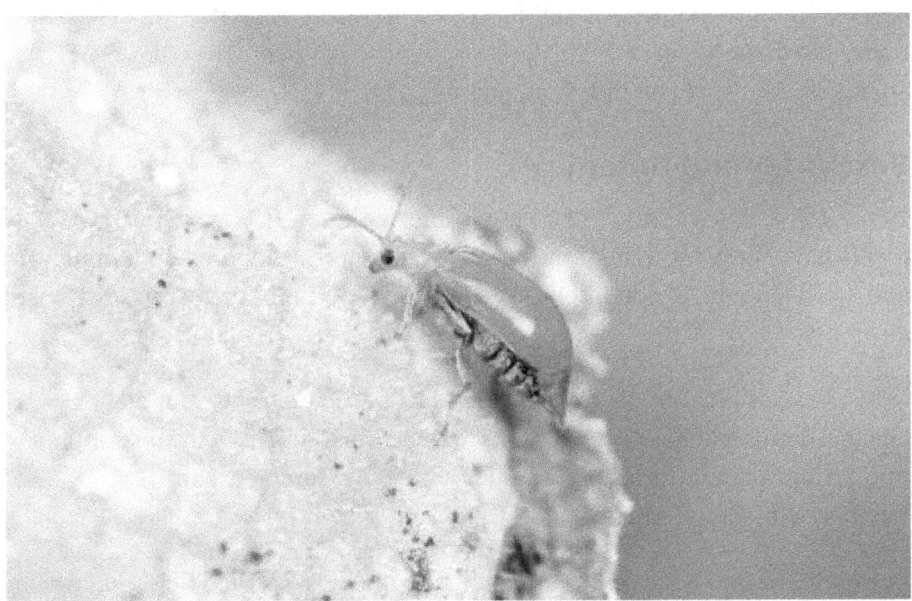

Also, the over use of insecticides have made many of these insects, immune to these pesticides. That is why in many parts of the world, larger quantities of arsenic was put in the pesticides by manufacturers who could not care less about the long-term very harmful effect of arsenic on the soil as well as on the consumer. This is the reason why it has been proven that rice produced in many parts of the world is not fit for consumption, unless you

---

[3] Cannot win any way you turn, can you?

want to suffer from diseases brought about through ingesting large quantities of arsenic.

So, that does not mean that you stop eating rice altogether. Look for organic brown rice. Do not buy polished rice. Look for wild rice. Start growing rice on your own – consider this to be a challenge – and you know that you are going to be eating healthy, poisonous pesticide free rice.

Also, lots of nitrogen fertilizer application made it possible for pests to flourish. So do not use any sort of chemical fertilizer, with lots of nitrogen in it. Try using organic manure and compost.

The common insect pests found in rice – apart from weevils – include rice bugs, and plant hoppers. Fungal diseases cause the plant growth getting stunted brown spots on the plant, leaf blot , etc.

Pesticides and Botanicals

Believe it or not, our unchecked use of pesticides on rice is overkill. Rice plants have been surviving four millenniums against flooding and drought, and adverse climatic conditions. They also have an inborn chemical defense against pests.

When we smother our plants with chemical pesticides, we are inducing changes in the plant, which prevents the chemical defenses from springing into action. That means our pesticides are encouraging pest attacks on vulnerable plants. Ironical, is not it.

In Cambodia and Vietnam, "companion plants" just for rice fields have been used as natural pesticides for thousands of years. These can come under the category of botanicals. These botanicals include extracts from plants and leaves or a mulch from the leaves, which, when spread over the surface of the soil is going to help retain the moisture, and facilitate the germination of the seeds. One of these plants is Chromolaena odorata also known as the Bitter Bush.

These leaves are also a natural fertilizer. Also, they prevent weeds from springing up, and of course they are an excellent pesticide.

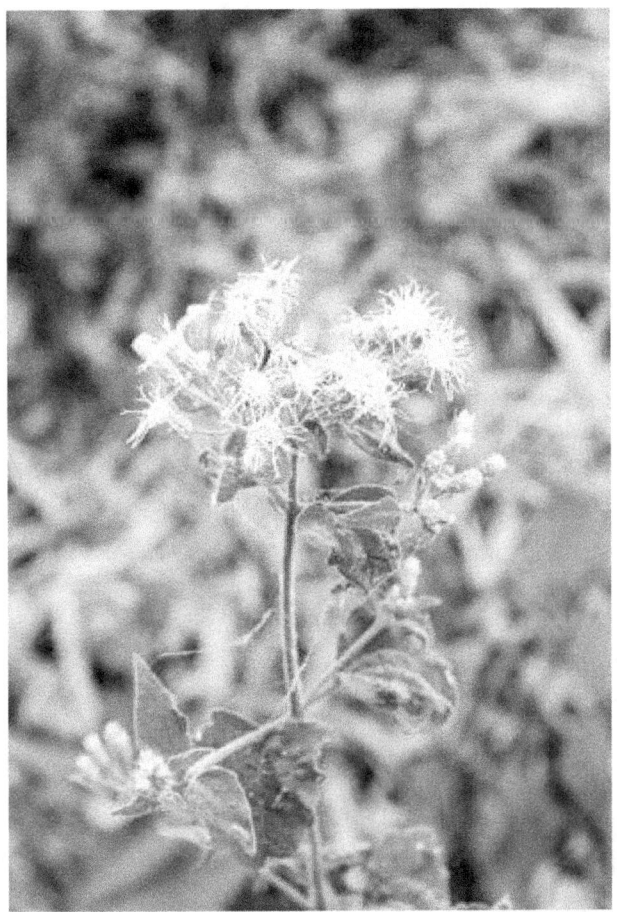

Bitter Bush

Popular Rice Cultivars

Apart from the world famous basmati, the popular Rice cultivars growing all over the world are Jereh and Buly grown in Indonesia, Jasmine rice, Japanese mochi rice and sake rice and floating rice, which can survive periodic flooding.

In the Indian subcontinent, the Rice cultivars are medium grained and long grained Patna rice, and the South Indian and Western Indian varieties, which include Ponni, Sona masuri, and Ambhemohar. This last named rice is considered to be a much in demand commodity, because it has a fragrance of the mango blossoms in bloom.

In America, you can get a basmati hybrid cultivar called Texmati! Other fragrant rice varieties include Patna rice, Nagpur Basmati and Vietnamese fragrant rice.

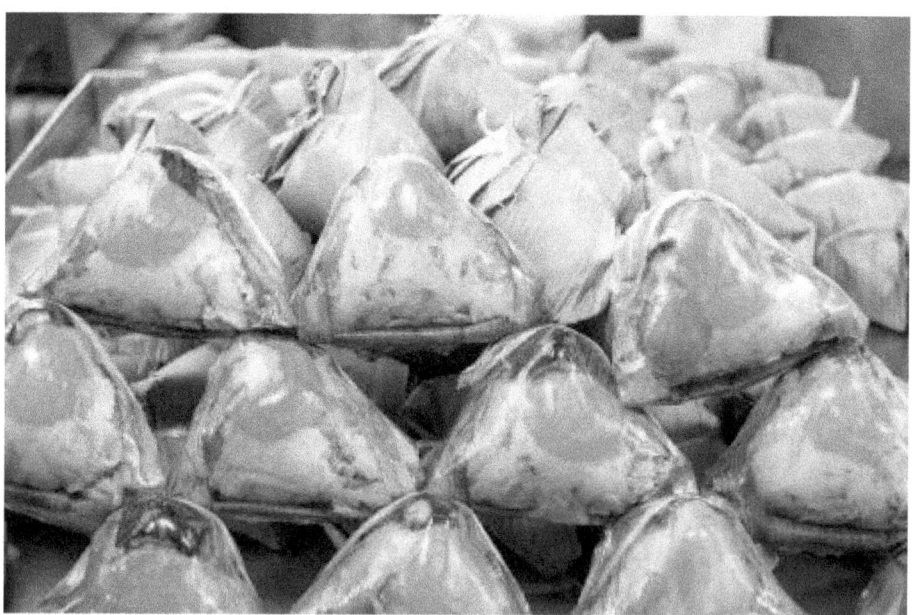

Traditional Rice dumplings known as zongzi are made by wrapping glutinous rice in a wrapping of bamboo leaves. They are a very popular part of Chinese fare.

Rice Dishes

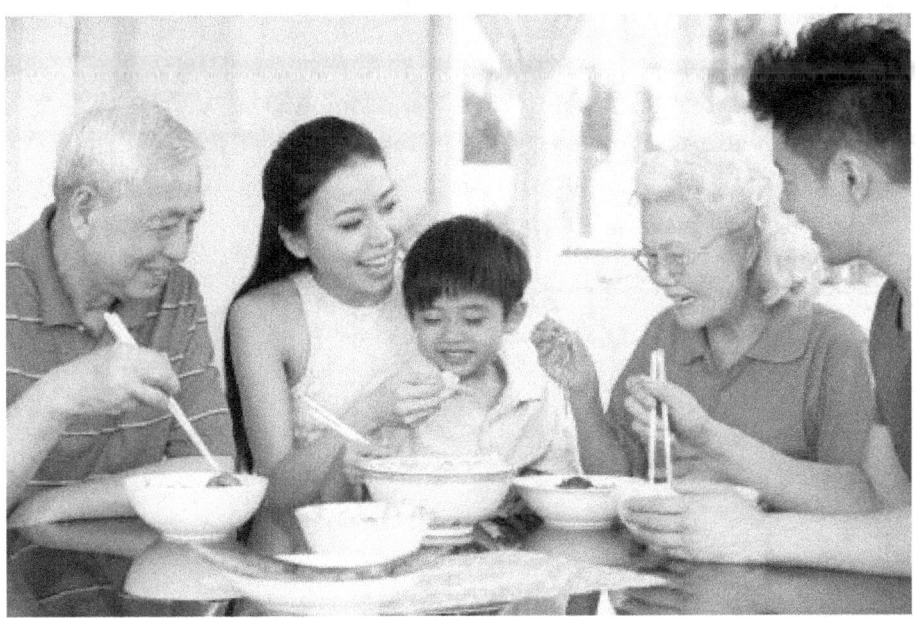

Rice is the staple diet of a large part of the world

Just imagine any cuisine in the world, ancient or modern, which does not have one particular dish made of rice. It can be steamed, baked, boiled, added to soups, dried, made into flour or can be used to any other creative and versatile use of which you can think. You can also use rice powder like beautiful Japanese geishas did, for ages,-as a face powder.

When I was living in South India as a kid, I used to see our neighbors preparing Dosai[4] batter for the next day's breakfast. This was a mixture of

---

[4] Here is a blog which I picked out if you are interested to try this traditional staple dish of the southern part of the Indian subcontinent and, incidentally, also a rage in many parts of the world today. Every Indian restaurant abroad is going to have this dish on its menu. The real name of this dish is Dosai, even though it is called Dosa.

http://www.rakskitchen.net/2014/05/dosa-recipe-south-indian-dosa.html

rice and lentils, – every family had its own traditional dosai batter recipe, which was a closely guarded secret – and I noticed that at that time that the proportions of the rice to the lentils as well as addition of different types of rice was quite enough to change the texture of the final product was definitely different.

That was because of the different rice flour additions. The Western equivalent of a Dosai is a crepe. The Huffington Post calls this particular dish one of the 10 dishes which you have to eat before you die. Naturally, the American barbecued steak makes this list!

If you find the names of the dals, just go to a shop where you get Indian ingredients. These are just cereals and lentils. Poha is flattened rice. Idli rice is shorter grained and parboiled. If you get it, well and good, otherwise just ask for parboiled rice.

Thanks to all the cereals and grains, this comes in one of the most nutritious food items list. You can stuff it with anything, including boiled potatoes or the filling of your choice.

Cooking Rice

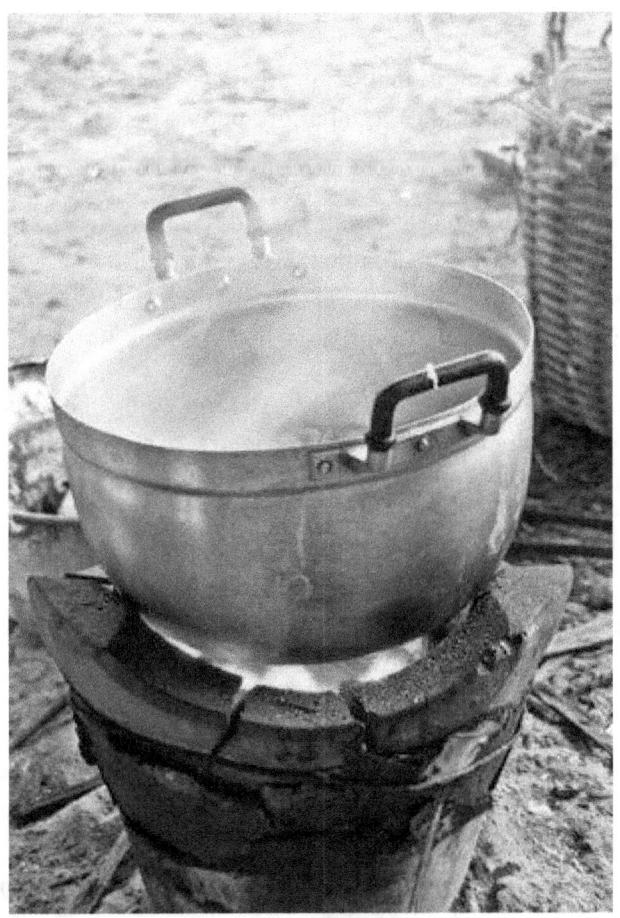

In many parts of the rural world, food is still being cooked outdoors on charcoal fires. The woman of the house may soon add wash rice to the water boiling in the Wok. For many people, even today, this is the only cooking pan used for cooking purposes. All the dishes are going to be made in this one pan and the family fed out of it, outdoors.

Rice needs to be washed a number of times before you cook it. That is because it has starch in it, and the nearest vestige of starch, left in the rice is going to cause stickiness between the grains during cooking.

When I was a youngster, I used to see my grandmother washing rice anywhere between 11 to 12 times before allowing it to soak for half an hour.

She never left this duty to the cook, because he would definitely take a shortcut and not bother about the water running clear before soaking.

Plain boiled rice is the traditional dish which is eaten throughout the world. 1 pound of rice is enough for 4 to 6 hungry people depending on their appetites.

The most in demand rice variety in the world, basmati, which literally means scent Of the Earth is available all over the world today. But how do you know the rice that you are eating is basmati? It has been packaged somewhere in Asia, possibly from Pakistan or from India.

Just take the grains of rice in your hand. All long grain rice is not basmati rice, whatever the exporter may say. You need to rub it vigorously over your Palm with your fingers, and then smell the palm of your hand.

Real basmati is going to give out a rich odor and fragrance of rice. When cooked, you should be able to smell it outside your door. The neighbors should come complaining "have you been cooking basmati rice again?" And then stay for dinner as the only way to be appeased for the crime of filling up the neighborhood with appealing and hungry making aromas.

Apart from these countries, you are also going to get top-quality rice – other varieties – from Myanmar, China, Korea, Bangladesh, Indonesia, Japan, Vietnam and Thailand – known all over the world for its delicious Jasmine rice – and the Philippines. 87% of the rice supplied globally, comes from these areas.

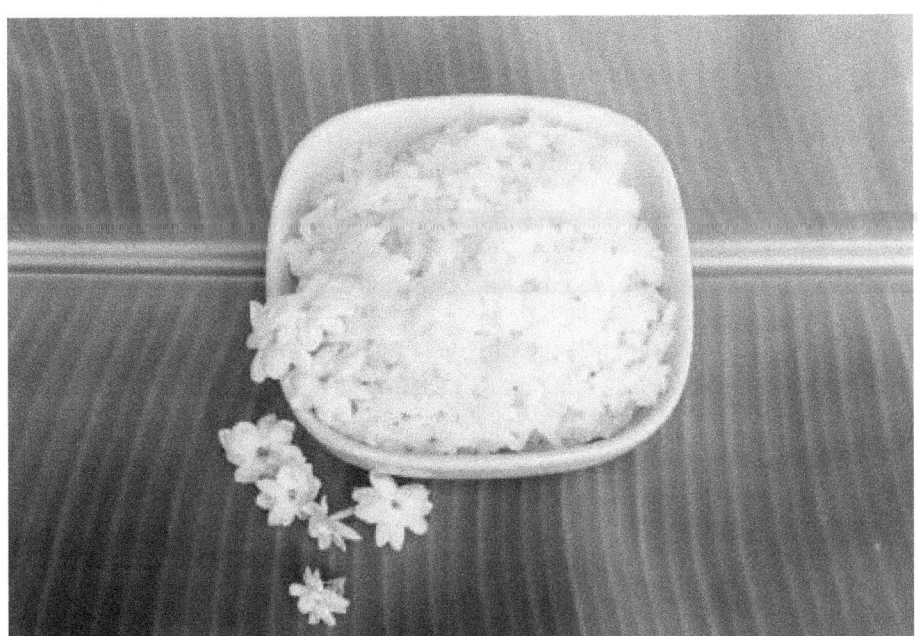

Jasmine rice

This rice if organically grown is worth the high cost you pay for it. It is also not going to have high quantities of arsenic, which are commonly used pesticides to control rice pests.

So now, I have this long grained rice in my hand. It may or may not be basmati. Basmati also comes in short grained varieties, did you know that? Rice comes in different colors ranging from Brown to red, purple, black and white. Different colors in rice grains depend on the variety and different colored pigments.

Once, when I was touring the Northeast region states of India on official duty, my boss told me that our hosts would be feeding us with native black rice. This was in 2004. All three of us juniors were told to eat the accompaniments politely, without too much of a fuss, because that would be rude.

Unfortunately, what we did not know that our Chief, had a rather malicious sense of humor. The accompaniment for those tiny caviar like grains of black rice was a paste made up of fish and Bhootjholokia – a red chilli with a Scoville heat units Rating of more than 1 million – about 900 times hotter than ordinary, and innocuous Tabasco sauce.

We literally Saw Ghosts[5] as the name suggested, at that time.

This once local chili has now gained international notoriety, but at that time it was just given to unsuspecting guests and subordinates who would then promise themselves to get even with The Chief , one fine day.[6]

So I did not manage to appreciate the taste, texture and quality of those native locally grown black grains of rice. But they are known to be a delicacy.

Now let us come back to cooking boiled rice traditionally.

The rice, which has been well washed and soaked – you can also wash the rice by leaving it in a deep pudding bowl under a briskly running tap for five – 10 minutes – is now ready for cooking.

Put the rice into a large quantity of boiling water. Many of us have the bad habit of putting the water on, on the stove and then dumping the rice into it. Not the proper way of cooking rice. The water has to be boiling. The water should be enough to allow all the grains to circulate freely when you are cooking.

Stir it gently and add one teaspoonful of salt. Here is one secret which I am going to tell you about how to whiten the grains of this boiling rice. I add half a teaspoonful of lemon juice at the same time when I am adding the salt.

---

[5] Especially I, who had taken a huge bite. The ensuing cavorting can easily be called the See a Ghost Dance along with noises. Chris and Mona just lay back on their seats, put their tongues out and panted, their eyes goggling like goldfish in a bowl. We had to drink down large quantities of yogurt to get rid of that burning sensation.

[6] We never did. He was too canny and wily a Fox.

Allow to boil, uncovered, for 7– 10 minutes. The rice is done when you test it between your finger and thumb sometime after seven minutes. You should not get a "granulated" feel. The center should be soft.

Pour off the water, and take the heat out of the rice by adding just enough of cold water to reduce the temperature until the rice is warm. This is going to stop the cooking process. You are also not going to get a rice pudding.

Strain through a colander, shake out on a dish and serve.

Do not throw the rice water away. It is called kanji (conjee) and I have really bad memories of it, especially as a youngster. I was 15, studying in a convent and suffering from amoebic dysentery. Sister Dometilla immediately put me on a rice water diet to get the supplements lost from the body back again. Try drinking boiled rice water with a little bit of salt in it, three times a day and nothing else. That is because She Knew that this was the best invalid diet and would set me going again.

It seems this barbarous practice is still being followed in many parts of the world, when children suffer from malnutrition or from amoebic dysentery! I managed to survive, but have not recovered from the weight loss incurred at the age of 15. Beats anorexia, anytime to give you a skeletal frame.

However, this rice water is nutritious and is often used to make rice porridge or rice gruel. This is done by adding more water to the rice until it disintegrates and then it can be done with salt.

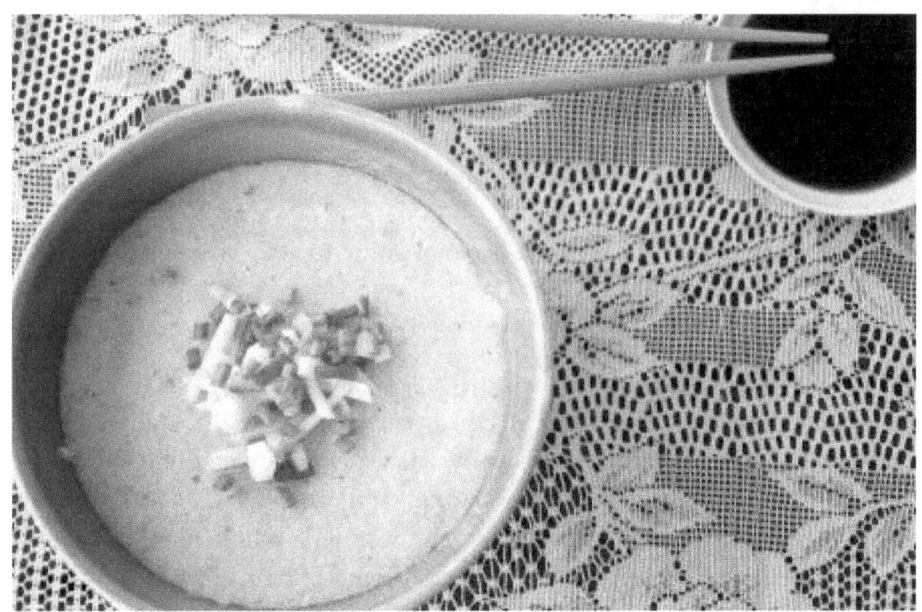

Rice porridge. It is considered to be a nutritious invalid diet as well as a healthy breakfast food.

Keep it away from me, please.

Even though I have heard, that this is eaten and enjoyed as a staple breakfast diet in many parts of the world.

With a little more effort, you can even cook lighter and starch free rice by washing again in cold water two or three times after cooking. Reheat by placing the rice covered in a moderate oven, or by washing with boiling water through a colander.

Rice can also be cooked in advance and completely cooled with cold water to stop the continued cooking and reheating as above.

Plain boiled rice is normally eaten with a gravy accompaniment. You can improve it by the addition of finely chopped onions, crisply fried in plenty of water and herbs.

Boiled rice always needs a generous quantity of water. You are going to remove the rice from the water when it is done. I have seen ladies waiting till the rice is tender and then throwing in a cup of cold water to halt the cooking process. That is also another way cool the rice down. They then serve the rice in a heated dish.

Reviving Overcooked Rice

Now this is one cooking technique, which everybody should know, especially if they have rice in large quantities on their daily menu. Overcooking normally happens when you put the rice in the water, and then forget that it is cooking away merrily. The end result is going to be broken grains of rice and possibly a starchy mess.

To revive this overcooked rice, run a lot of cold water in a colander or sieve until nearly cold. Then drain well and warm, covered, in a low oven or with hot water.

Always remember to use fresh water when you are cooking rice. That means you are not going to use the water in which it had been soaked for half an hour. But if you need to use the soaking water, remember to strain it through fine muslin cloth so that any sort of impurities left over after washing can be removed in this last straining.

Steamed Rice

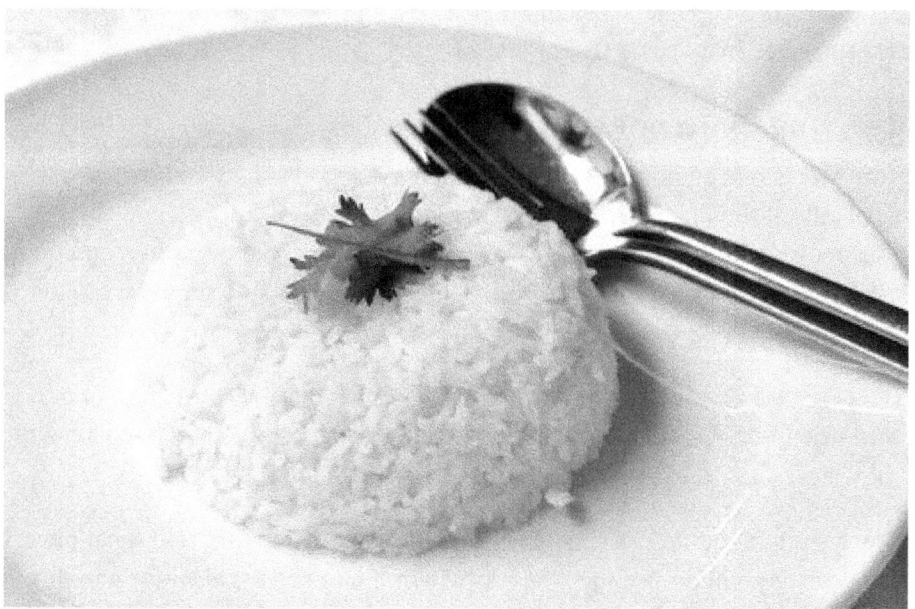

Rice is normally cooked by steaming in many South and Southeast Asian countries and the moistening is going to vary according to the cooking vessel, the amount of heat used, the type of rice and even the time of the year.

Begin with salted water with a dash of lemon juice. This water should rise 1 – 1 ¼ inches above the uncooked rice. The water content is going to be less if the quantities are even smaller.

Boil, stirring for one minute, cover with a tight fitting lid and reduce the heat. When the water has been absorbed, you can test the rice by withdrawing a few grains from the center. If more cooking is necessary, – i.e. the rice grain does not feel soft at the center when you rub a piece between the thumb and forefinger – sprinkle in just a tablespoonful of so of water.

Close the lid, then steam on a gentle heat, repeating the sprinkling water process until the rice is tender. After a few sessions, you are going to judge the amount of water needed. When this is done, place the rice in a cool place for 10 minutes before serving.

Traditional Pilavs and Biriyanis

Apart from boiled rice and steamed rice, any rice, which has an addition of nuts, spices, dry fruit, vegetables, and meat can be traditionally called a pilav or a biryani. Both of them are different dishes. The Spanish paella is the Spanish version of the Persian pilav.

Here is the traditional recipe for

Savory Pilau With Chicken

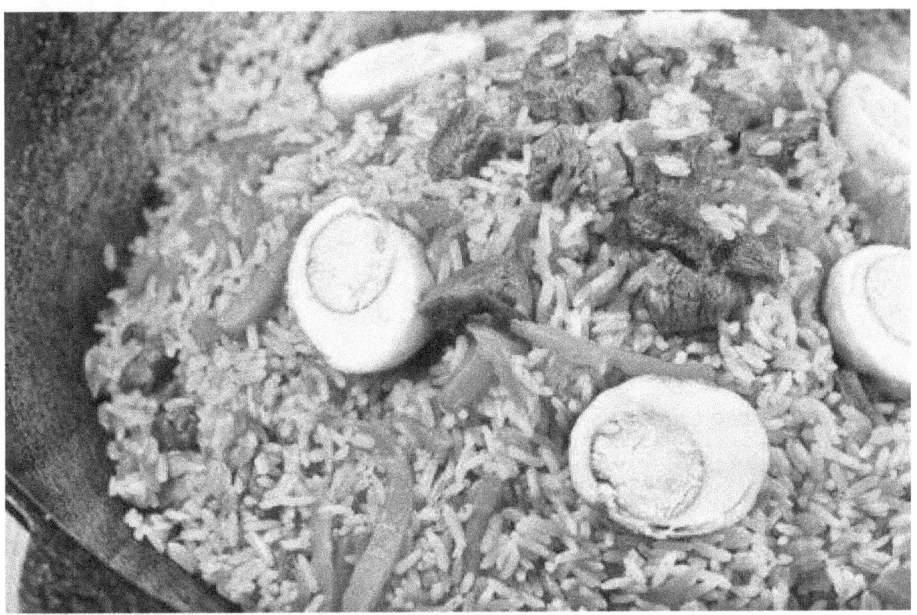

This particular pilau seems to have slices of carrots added to it!

For this you need **half a pound of rice, two medium onions grated, 3 ounces of butter, 2 pounds of roasting chicken, one integrated green ginger, 6 tablespoons yogurt, salt to taste, six – eight cloves of garlic, ¼ teaspoon cumin seeds, minced, one teaspoonful of freshly ground black pepper, five cardamoms, ground, two broken bay leaves, ¼ teaspoon nutmeg, 1 inch splintered stick of cinnamon, one large minced pimento, one tablespoonful of chopped mint, one – two, dried or fresh red chilies roasted lightly and seeded.**

Pieces of lemon and onions, cut into rings for garnish

Soak the rice in cold water for one hour. This is normally made on festive occasions in the East, and that is why the best quality rice is chosen. Choose long grain rice, which it does not stick. When cooked this rice is going to give out a fragrant aroma of cooked to perfection rice, perhaps basmati.

Prepare the spices. Dice the bird in eight pieces. Drain the rice and leave to dry. Brown the cumin seeds and then the grated onions in the butter until all the moisture has dried up.

Put the chicken in and fry it over medium heat. Add the ginger and cook for a further five minutes. Now add a few tablespoons whole of the yogurt, season with salt and on low heat until the chicken is soft and tender. This is going to take about 35 minutes. All the moisture will have dried by then.

Add the garlic for aroma, and moisten with even more yogurt. Add the bay leaves, black pepper, cinnamon, cardamoms, nutmeg, mint and pimento

Put in the rice and fry for another five – six minutes. Add the water to cover the rice by 1 ¼ inches and stir well.

Add the chopped chilies. Bring just to boiling point than cook over the lowest possible heat until the rice has been cooked completely. Give it the last steaming in a low oven are over an asbestos mat on the top of the stove for 12 minutes.

Leave for five minutes in a warm atmosphere, uncover and serve with wedges of lemon and round slices of onion.[7]

---

[7] Traditionally in ancient Persia, these pilavs were cooked in copper utensils and brought straight to the feasting table. Unfortunately, the prices of copper utensils today are prohibitive, so I am always on the lookout for ancient utensils which are being discarded by people who do not know their real value.

Biryani

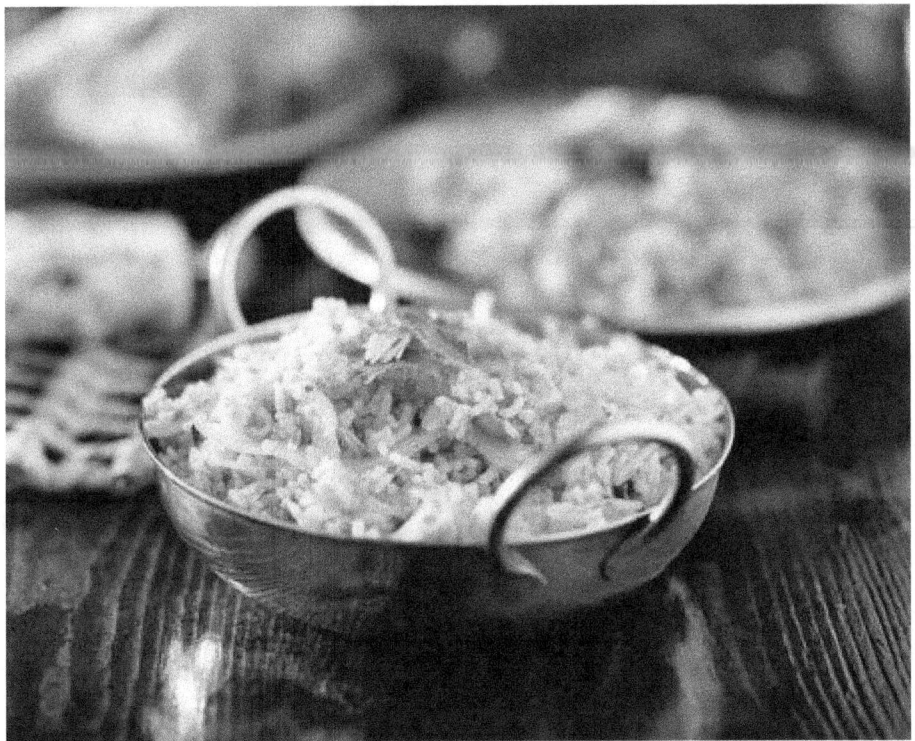

The biryani you eat in a number of Indian restaurants all over the world today are a shadow of the real thing made traditionally. These dishes are mass-produced in a hurry, to feed hungry customers, who think that the heavily spiced, greasy mixture in front of them is the real thing. It is not.

Here is the traditional recipe of the original biryani, which originated somewhere in Central Asia centuries ago. Invaders and explorers took the recipe of biryani along with them to the lands they conquered.

There are many kinds of traditional biryani. The pakka biryani is normally made with cooked rice. The kacha biryani is named after the uncooked rice and the katcha-pakka variety is naturally going to be made of parboiled rice.

Different techniques are used for each preparation. The final dish is always going to be vividly colored and spiced substantially.

The original Zarebriyan biryani, also known as the biryani – Palau is distinguished from other rice preparations in three ways.

It is going to be colored or flavored with turmeric or saffron if you can afford it. It is going to have cumin and coriander seed, whole peppercorns and large black cardamoms in it.

Other aromatics are going to vary, according to availability, taste and choice. This particular biryani is richer than other pilaus because of the amount of butter which you are going to use in it. Finally, you are going to put twice as much meat or fish as rice in it.

Traditional Biryani – spiced Meat Pilau

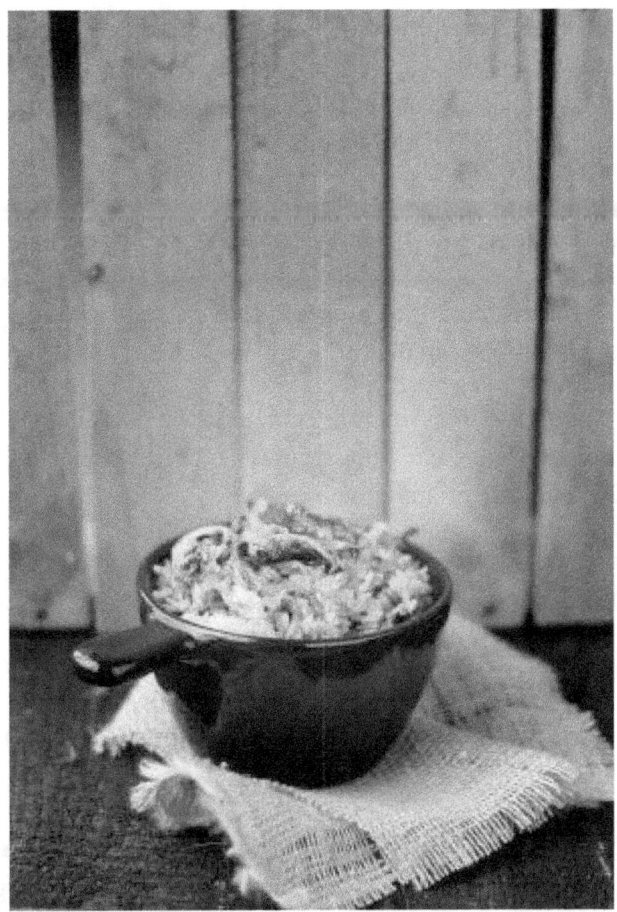

Biryani is always accompanied with a gravy.

For this you need one and a half pounds of lamb, pork or beef, one small handful of parsley and coriander leaves, 2 inches of green ginger, one teaspoonful of salt, 3 inches of cinnamon, one green pimento, two green chilies, eight large crushed cardamoms, 10 cloves, 4 ounces of butter, 1 pound of rice, one tablespoonful of turmeric, 3 tablespoons full of ground coriander seed, one tablespoonful of ground cumin, half a teaspoonful of cayenne, one tablespoonful of whole peppercorns, 4 ounces of raisins, washed, 10 crushed cloves of garlic, six large onions, and 2 ounces of blanched almonds.

A biryani is always made with a broth. The meat is going to be used here, and you can use a few bones as well. Cover by about 4 inches with cold water and add shredded coriander leaves, chopped green ginger, salt, half of the cinnamon, the pimento and the chilies.

Boiled ones, skim, and simmer until the meat is tender. This is going to take one – three hours, according to the type of meat along with the cut and size.

You can cut the meat into 2 inch pieces before or after cooking. Drain the meat and allow to dry. Strain the broth and preserve.

Place the cardamoms, cloves, and the remaining cinnamon crushed a bit, in a Muslin cloth bag. Heat some butter and fry the rice with ¾ each quantity of the turmeric, cumin, coriander, and cayenne.

When translucent, add the muslin bag, the peppercorns, washed raisins, crushed garlic, and enough of water to cover by 1 ½ inches. Season with salt and bring to a boil. Lower heat and simmer.

Meanwhile, melt a little butter in a large frying pan and cook the meat of with the remaining turmeric, coriander, cumin and cayenne until a rich brown in color.

Quarter the onions and separate into layers, then fry fast until they are colored, but still crisp. That means the onions are going to be slightly undercooked. Add the almonds, mix well and keep warm.

When the rice is almost cooked, uncover and quickly add the contents of the frying pan, scraping up all the butter and the crusty part. Mix the rice and the meat well and cover.

Raise the heat very high for a few seconds then give it the steaming treatment for 10 minutes in a moderate oven, leaving aside for three – four minutes before serving.

Remember that this dish was made in a land, where spices and dried fruit were very common. But it took a really long time to prepare. That is why this dish was eaten traditionally just on festive occasions. On special occasions or on feast days, the whole tribe would gather around the planter of biryani and dig in with the right hand.[8] Eating from the same platter was a symbolic act of the brotherhood of the tribe.

Even today, in many parts of the East and Central Asia, biryani made the traditional way has to be served – in the dish in which it was cooked – during any joyous celebration or festive occasion.

---

[8] This activity may bring up a vision of Barbaric and savage Central Asian invaders eating in a hearty, noisy and gluttonous fashion, but these peoples and tribes were known to have amazingly dainty and gracious eating habits and very cultured table manners. This was documented by Western visitors to their cities and towns in the 13th and 14th centuries. In fact, the French court learned neat and dainty table manners and table etiquette from these "heathenish and barbaric lands" through warriors who had gone there on the holy Crusades. Only the tips of two fingers and the thumb were used to convey food to the mouth. The rest of the hand would stay completely clean. Even today the same table manners are practiced at home and in public.

Brown Rice and Polished Rice

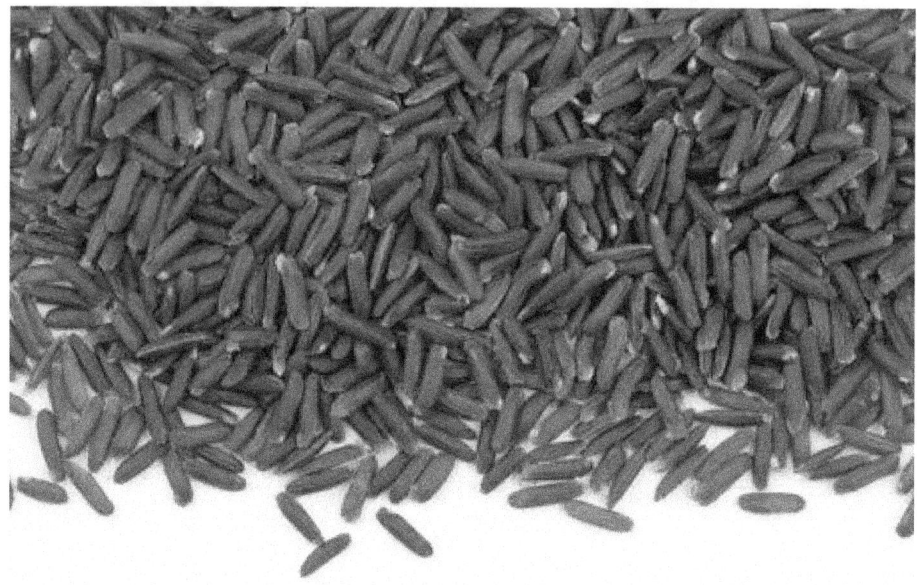

This is a species of harvested brown rice from Thailand. Polishing is going to turn it white.

Harvested rice seeds have to be milled first, so that the chaff is removed. Now days, people use rice hullers to do this, when once they used to "winnow" by hand, in huge woven trays.[9]

The rice which you are going to get now is Brown Rice. If this is organically grown, this is the healthiest rice, which you can obtain. However, because we cannot resist making national things even more unpalatable, we have to subject it to processing and polishing. Thus, we effectively make sure that all the nutrients are diminished significantly.

---

[9] If you want to see how that is done, even today in many parts of the world, here is the URL –

http://www.learnnc.org/lp/editions/vietnam-farming/458

The polished Rice, which you buy on your supermarket shelf is going to be white rice created by removing the bran through continuous milling that means that the rest of the germ, and the husk has been removed. This white rice is going to keep longer, but it is not going to have all the nutrients which Brown rice could give you.

Brown rice eaten regularly prevented beriberi down the ages. White rice has absolutely no intention of doing so, because it has been powdered, painted and polished. It looks so attractive, but it is definitely not going to improve your health. That is because the polishing process was done with glucose and talc!

You mean, you say, you have been eating talc, the same talc , which you use as a deodorant? Well, the answer is yes. Along with glucose, used by manufacturers and rice packagers to give your rice a pretty shine and allowing it to last longer.

Real unpolished rice, if you are lucky to get it is normally preserved for about one year, before it is sent out into the market. I remember my grandmother, opening up one of these treasured sacks, and telling us kids to wash the rice.

We were immediately rather horrified. There were weevils in the rice. We were not going to eat anything with horrors, weevils in it. But that, she told us, was the sign that this rice was the original stuff and had gone through one season of the year, when weevils got a chance to grow in the rice.

So the rice was washed very, very carefully, because after all, father intended to make his famous and delicious Pilau for Sunday lunch. And the ensuing dish was marvelous, with lots of spices, and I remember with added chicken fat, and pieces of chicken fried, and spread all over the pulao, in one of his creative culinary innovations.

So if your rice has weevils in it, you know, it is the real thing in its matured form and this maturing enhances the taste, flavor, fragrance and texture of the end product.

You may find packaged rice in your supermarket, giving you information on the package that you should not wash the rice before cooking. That is because this rice has already been subjected to the polishing process with nutrients added to it. Do you consider this sensible? First natural nutrients are removed by these enterprising young gentlemen. After that, they add nutrients to the rice, which is going to wash off, according to their instructions. Some even have water soluble nutrients, coating the surface of the rice.

I am rather chary of such innovations, and wonder about their long-term and possibly detrimental effect they would have on the health of a regular consumer of such processed, preserved and prinked up rice.

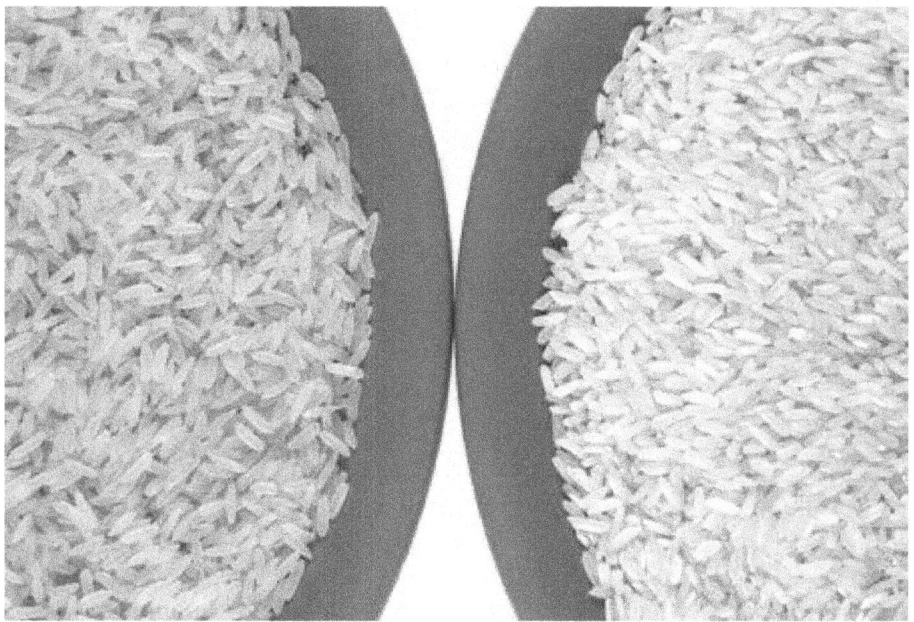

The yellow colored rice on the left is parboiled.

In many parts of the world, especially in Africa, rice is subjected to steaming while it is still in its brown rice form. That means all the nutrients are going to shift from the outer husk and get absorbed by the grain. So this parboiled rice, even though yellowish in color is definitely going to be far superior in the matter of nutrients than any other available rice, which has been subject to processing and polishing.

The best thing about this parboiled rice is that it is not going to stick to your cooking pan, when you are cooking it. That is because it has already been cooked halfway and also has been subjected to a drying process. That means the cooking time is going to be shorter for this type of rice.

Talc processed rice is banned in many of the countries all over the world, and in the USA, this process is on its way out. The rice bran can be heated to produce rice oil, which is used extensively in Japan to make traditional daikon horseradish pickles called Takuwan.

If you are suffering from gluten intolerance, try using rice flour, which is an excellent substitute for gluten laden wheat flour.

Eating uncooked rice seeds, just like any other cereals is not advised at all. Remember that this staple food may be rich in protein, but eating rice just on its own is not going to give you the full supplement of nutrients your body needs to keep functioning in a healthy fashion. That is why rice is always accompanied with meat, beans, seeds, vegetables, nuts, or any other culinary accompaniment you wish.

Conclusion

This book has introduced you to the magic of rice, that gift of the gods, which has fed millions down the ages. If you have grown your own rice, and have felt that sense of achievement, here are some more tips on how you can save the seeds for next season's sowing.

The average and proven yield of rice per hectare is anywhere between 7 tons to 10 tons, even though claims have been made for record harvests of 19 tons, up to 22.4 tons per hectare through genetically modified plants.

But we are not talking in tons or hectares, because we are just ordinary run of the mill gardeners with a limited farming space or just our own little backyard! So we are going to preserve our rice harvest by selecting all the healthy plant panicles. After the grains have been sorted out, choose the clean grains without any blemish or fault.

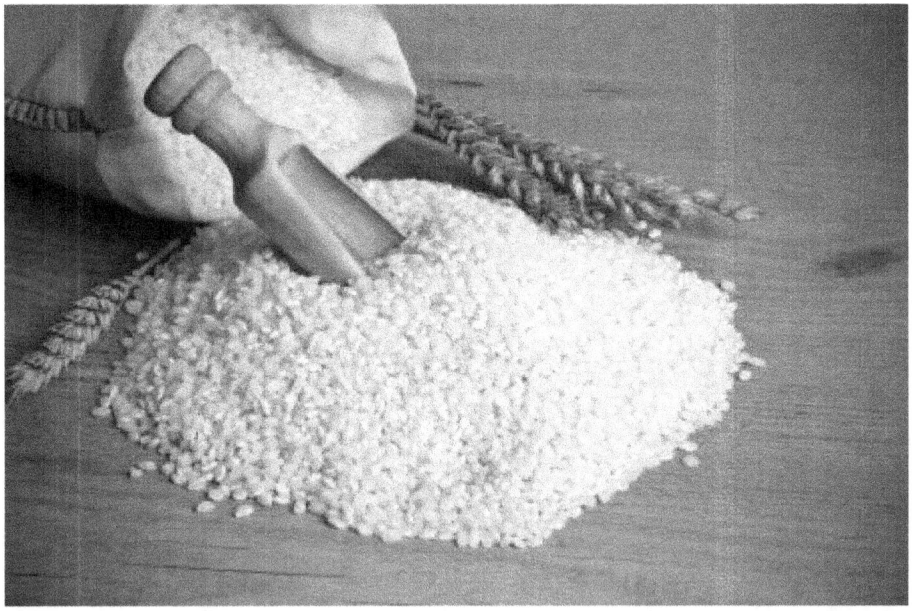

These seeds are kept in boxes or containers, which are airtight. Do not place them in polythene bags or in gunnysacks. Did you know that USD22 billion worth of rice harvest is going to waste every year in a number of countries in Asia, because their governments could not bother about providing better storage facilities to the farmers?

It has been calculated by researchers that this grain was enough to feed *10 million people every year*.

So as one says, no one need go hungry again, but mankind cannot be taught sense and reason, or bother to learn something for the benefit of his hungry brethren, just because he could not care less.

This criminal wastage is on par with the dumping of a bumper wheat harvest into the sea because the farmers did not know way to store it, how to sell it and what to do with it. That was in the 60s and matters have not changed since then. Believe it or not, this was in a developed country. So if that is the situation there, what would one expect in Third World and still developing countries.[10]

Traditionally, rice was preserved in earthenware pots. The pots were sealed, both on the inside and on the outside with cooking oil. After that it was put in the sun so that the oil would close the pores of the pot. After a day of sunning, the pot would be washed and dried thoroughly before the seeds were placed in them. The container would then be closed with an airtight lid and sealed with a cloth, tied with a rope and placed in the dry cellar.

---

[10] This is also the reason why I have seen totally disgruntled farmers dumping their bumper crop of potatoes and tomatoes on the roadside for anyone to pick and take back home. [I see this every two – three years in my region which is agriculture oriented.] They have no transport facilities to send their harvest to other States. The state government could not care less.

And when other parts of the country is starved of high in demand potatoes and tomatoes, they are squashed underfoot by people in our region, walking on the roads.

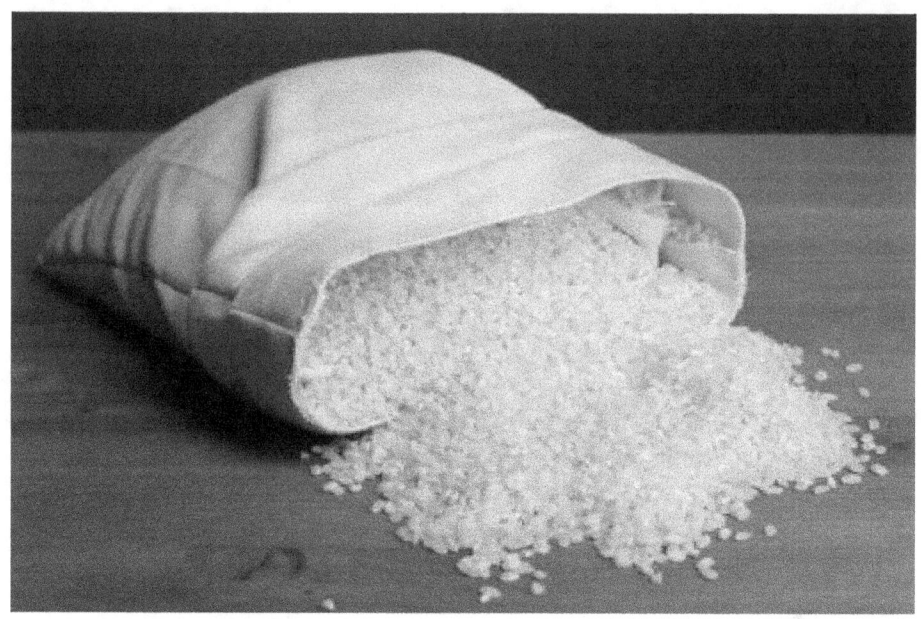

Cloth bags are still being used in many parts of the world to store rice.

The container was usually filled up to the brim. This makes sense, because an empty space can allow insects. That is because there is oxygen in the pot.If you do not have enough of seeds, fill up the rest of the pot with very dry sand and natural insect repellents like dried neem leaves. And then close the lid and make it airproof.

Believe it or not, I saw one of my acquaintances putting naphthalene balls in the storage area where she stored food items. This specimen comes under the stubborn fool category who does not understand that chemicals like naphthalene should be kept away from food items. Also, just imagine all that gentle fragrance of high quality rice being subjected to the harsh and unpleasant odor of naphthalene.

These containers have to be replaced on a stand or a shelf high up from the ground so that their content does not get damaged or damp.

Remember that High quality Good seeds properly stored today, means a good harvest tomorrow. So allow the good plant rice to enter your life, Live Long and Prosper!

Author Bio

Dueep Jyot Singh is a Management and IT Professional who managed to gather Postgraduate qualifications in Management and English and Degrees in Science, French and Education while pursuing different enjoyable career options like being an hospital administrator, IT,SEO and HRD Database Manager/ trainer, movie , radio and TV scriptwriter, theatre artiste and public speaker, lecturer in French, Marketing and Advertising, ex-Editor of Hearts On Fire (now known as Solstice) Books Missouri USA, advice columnist and cartoonist, publisher and Aviation School trainer, ex-moderator on Medico.in, banker, student councilor ,travelogue writer … among other things!

One fine morning, she decided that she had enough of killing herself by Degrees and went back to her first love -- writing. It's more enjoyable! She already has 48 published academic and 14 fiction- in- different- genre books under her belt.

When she is not designing websites or making Graphic design illustrations for clients , she is browsing through old bookshops hunting for treasures, of which she has an enviable collection – including R.L. Stevenson, O.Henry, Dornford Yates, Maurice Walsh, De Maupassant, Victor Hugo, Sapper, C.N. Williamson, "Bartimeus" and the crown of her collection- Dickens "The Old Curiosity Shop," and so on… Just call her "Renaissance Woman") - collecting herbal remedies, acting like Universal Helping Hand/Agony Aunt, or escaping to her dear mountains for a bit of exploring, collecting herbs and plants and trekking.

Check out some of the other JD-Biz Publishing books

Gardening Series on Amazon

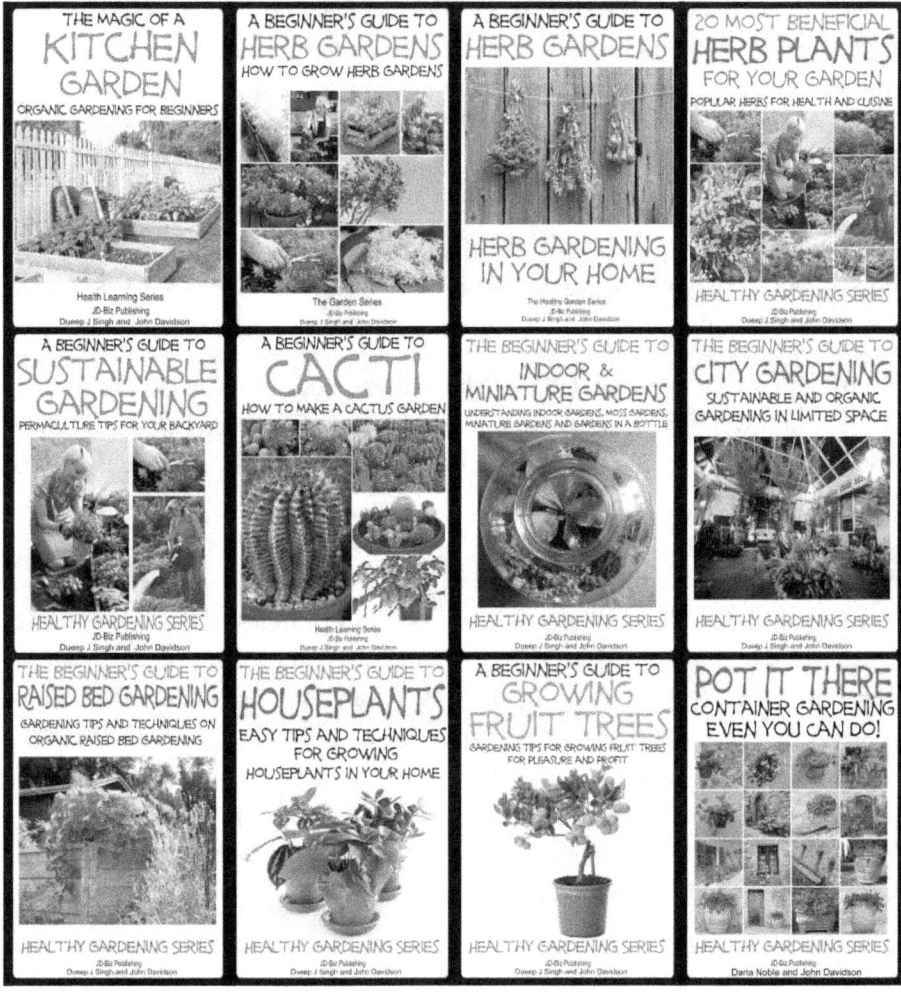

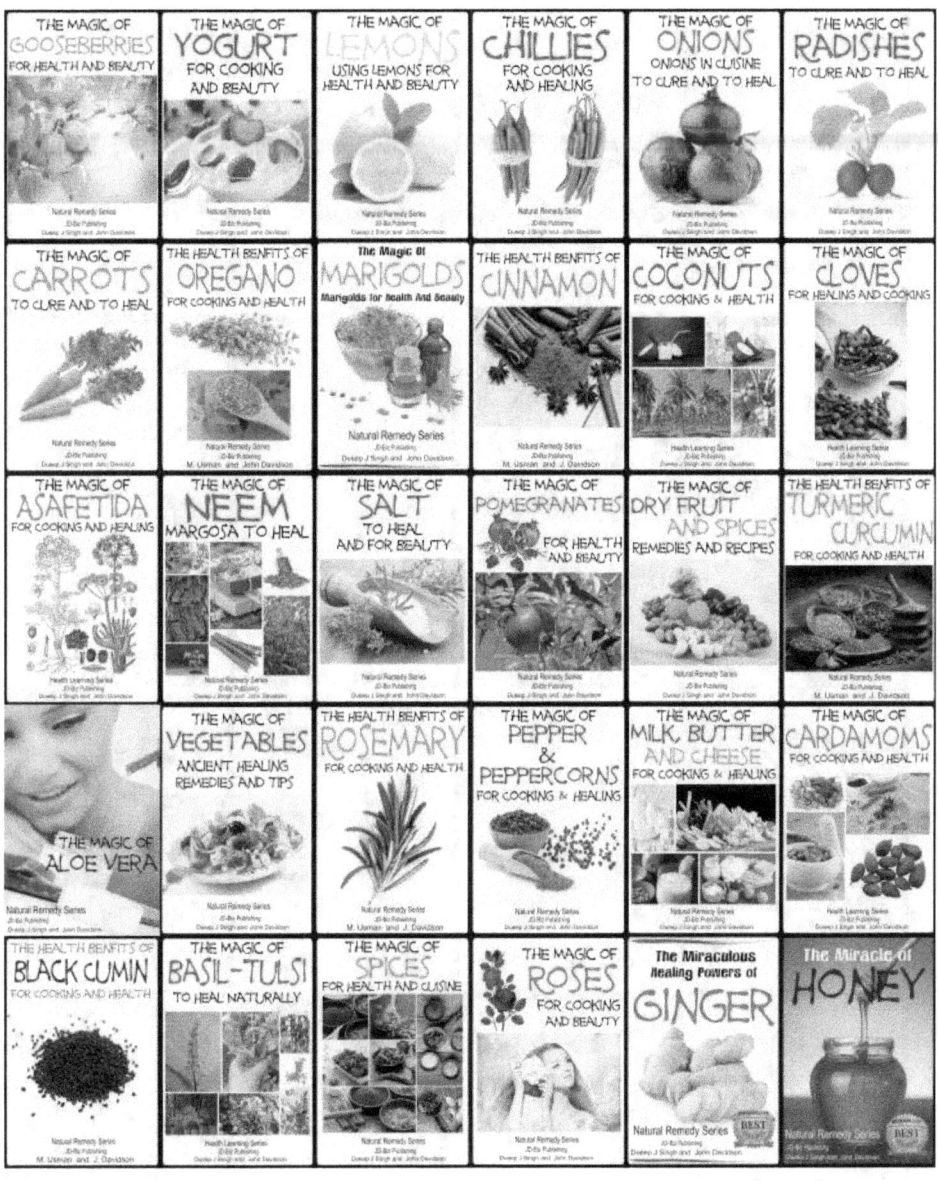

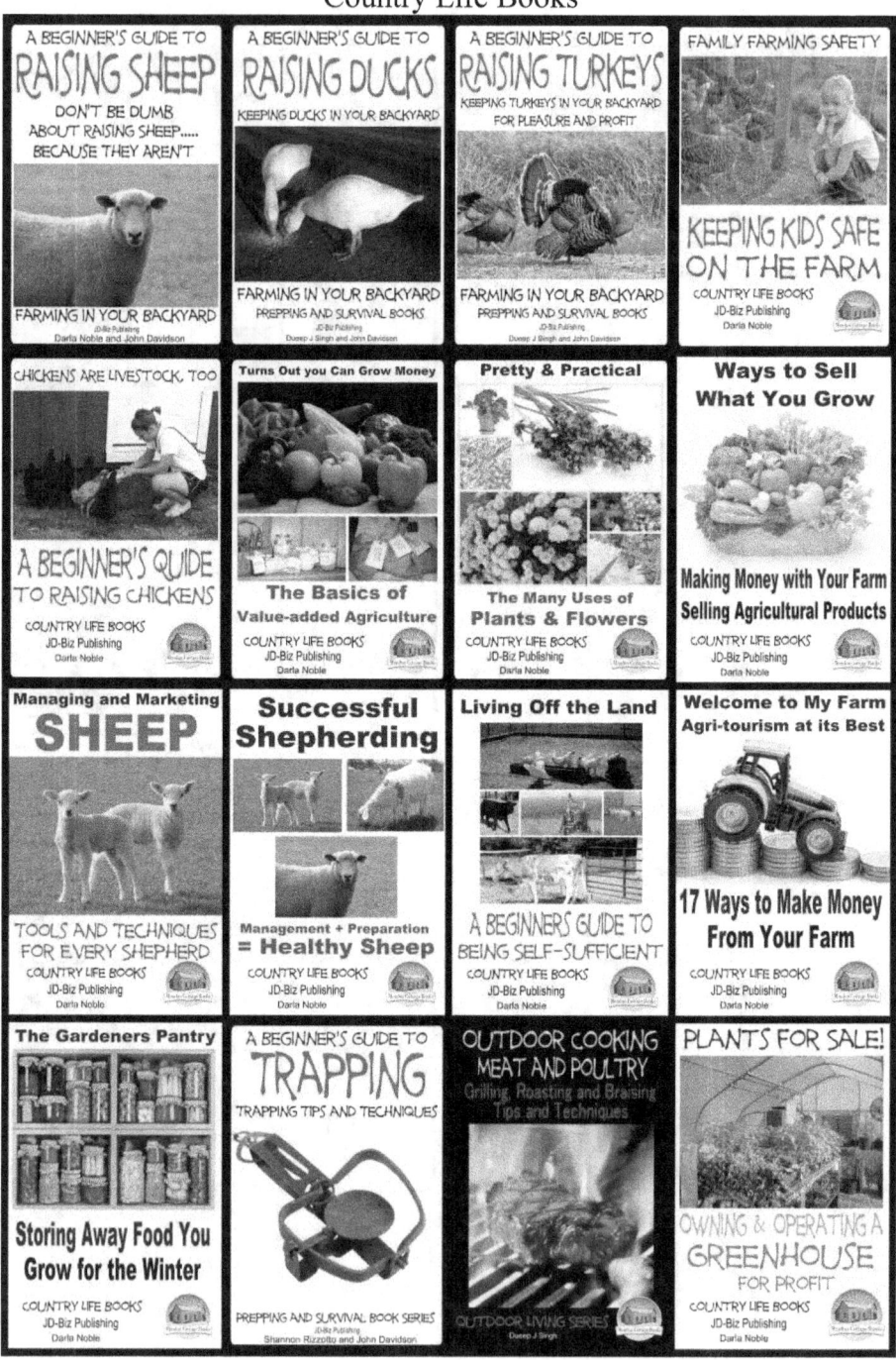

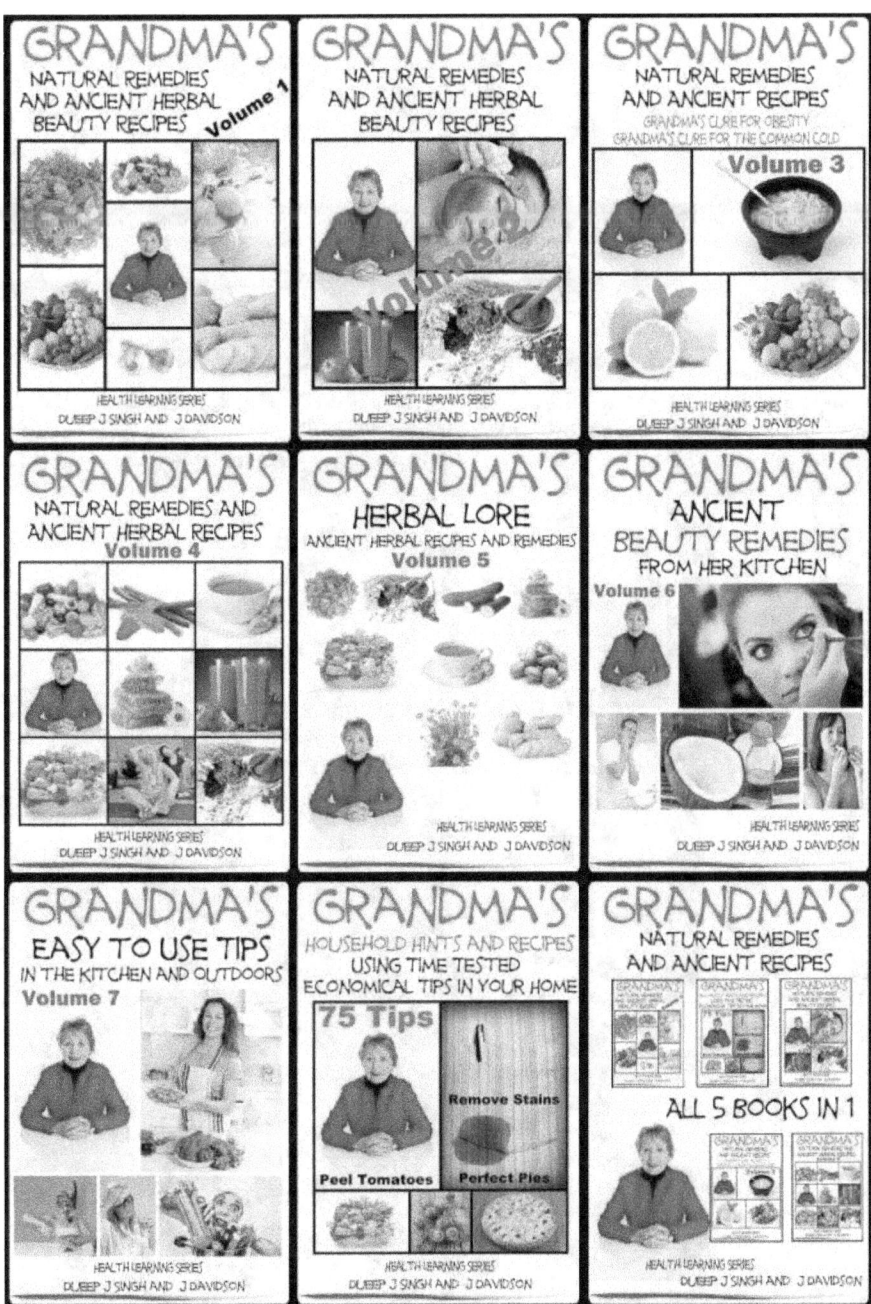

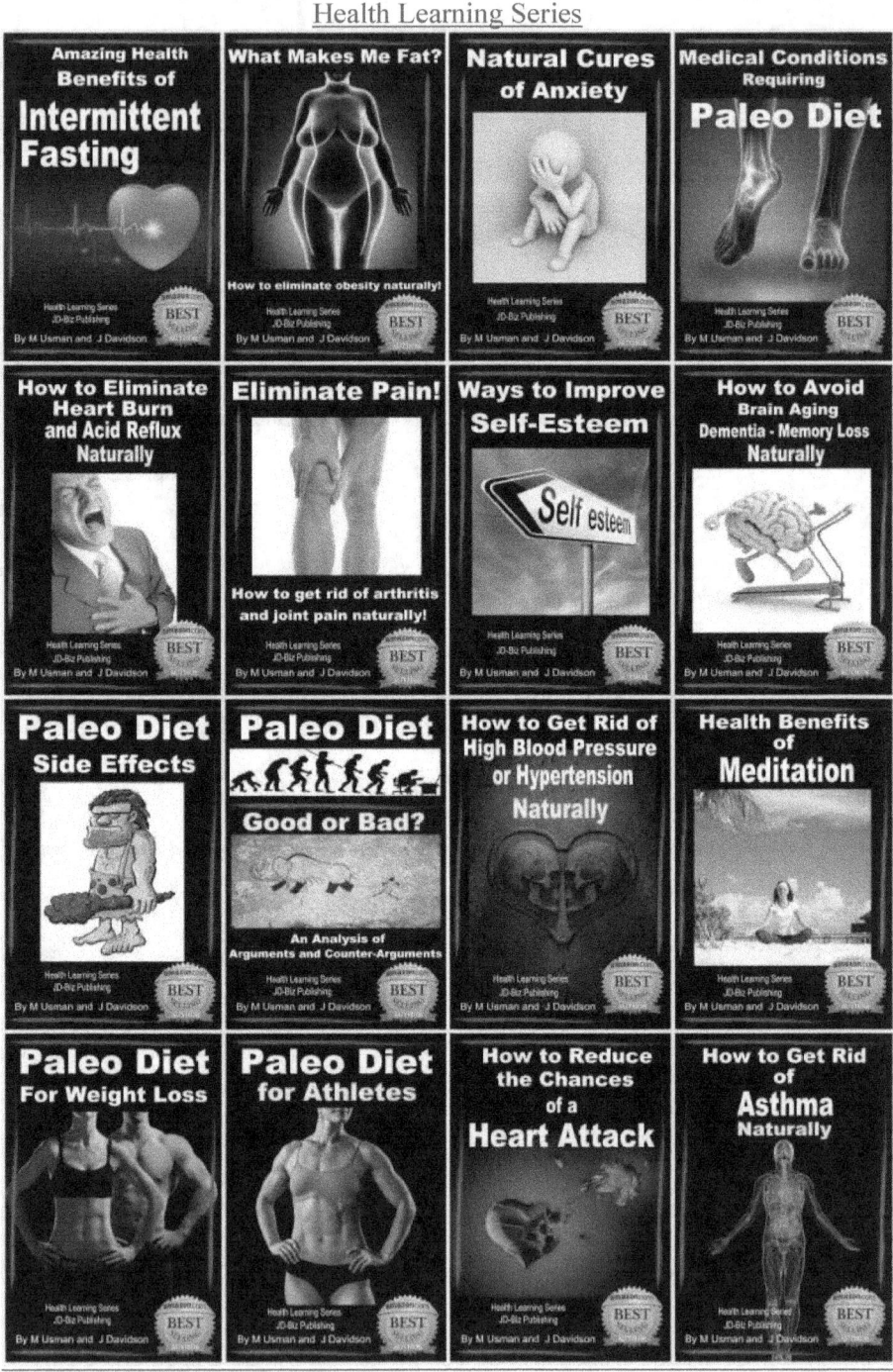

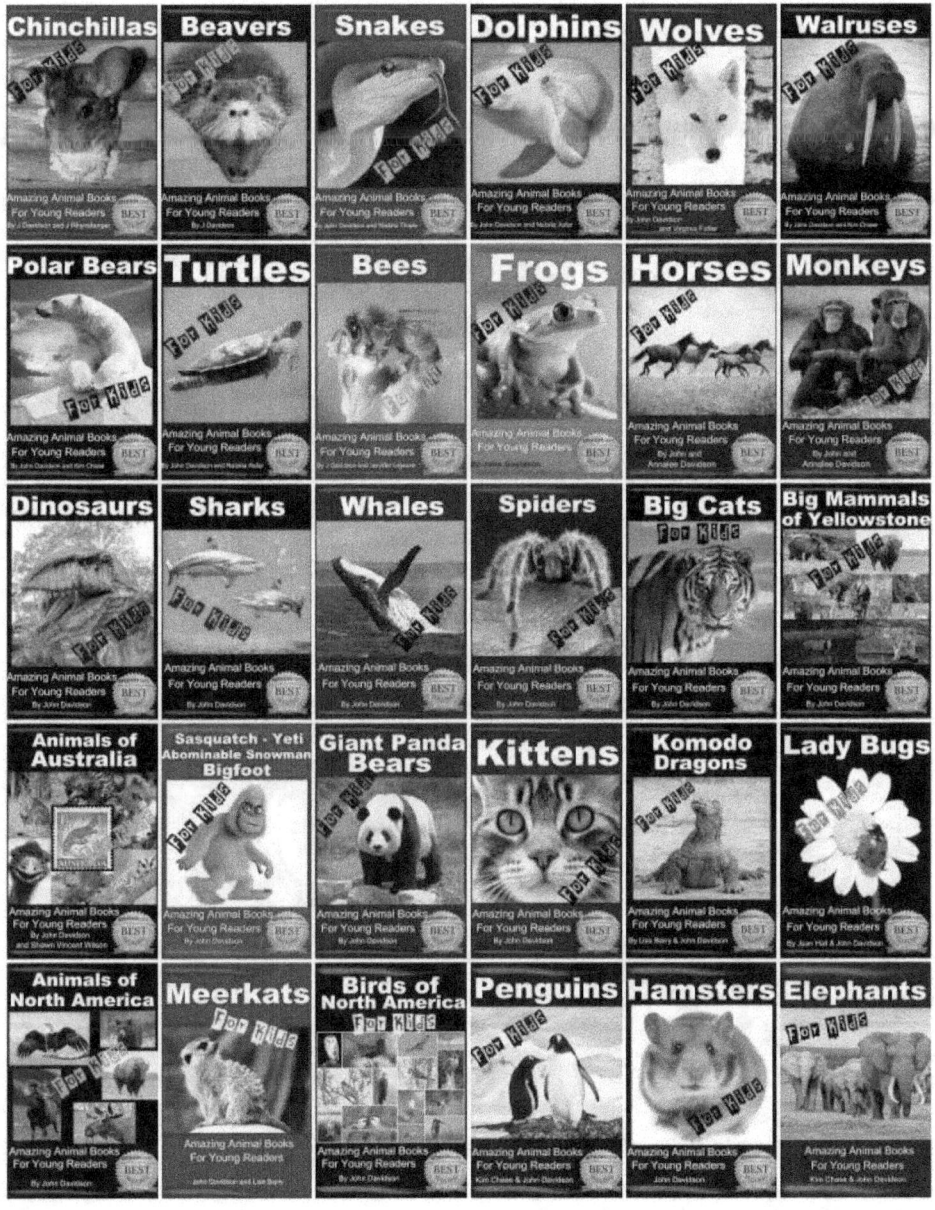

Learn To Draw Series

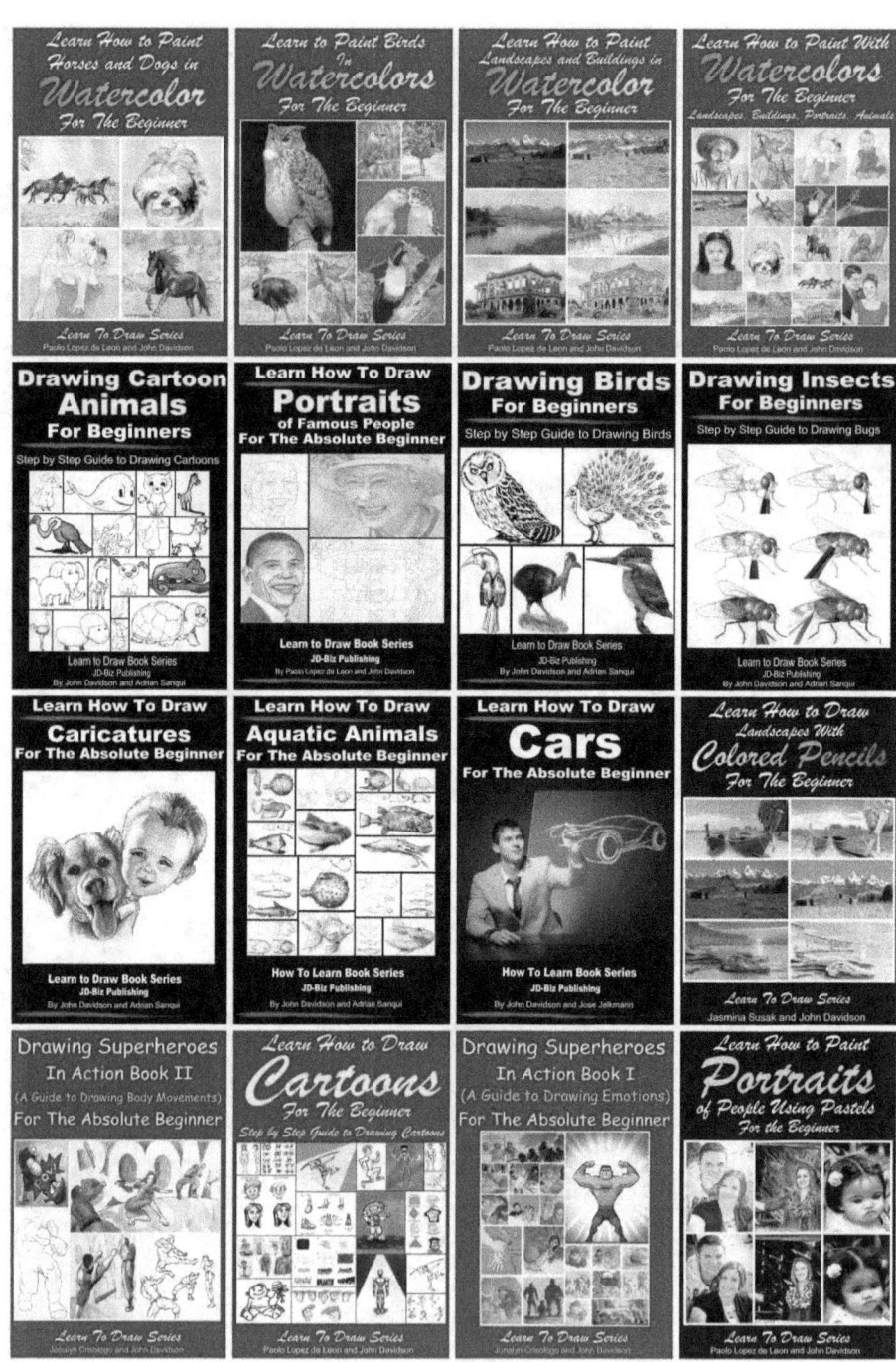

How to Build and Plan Books

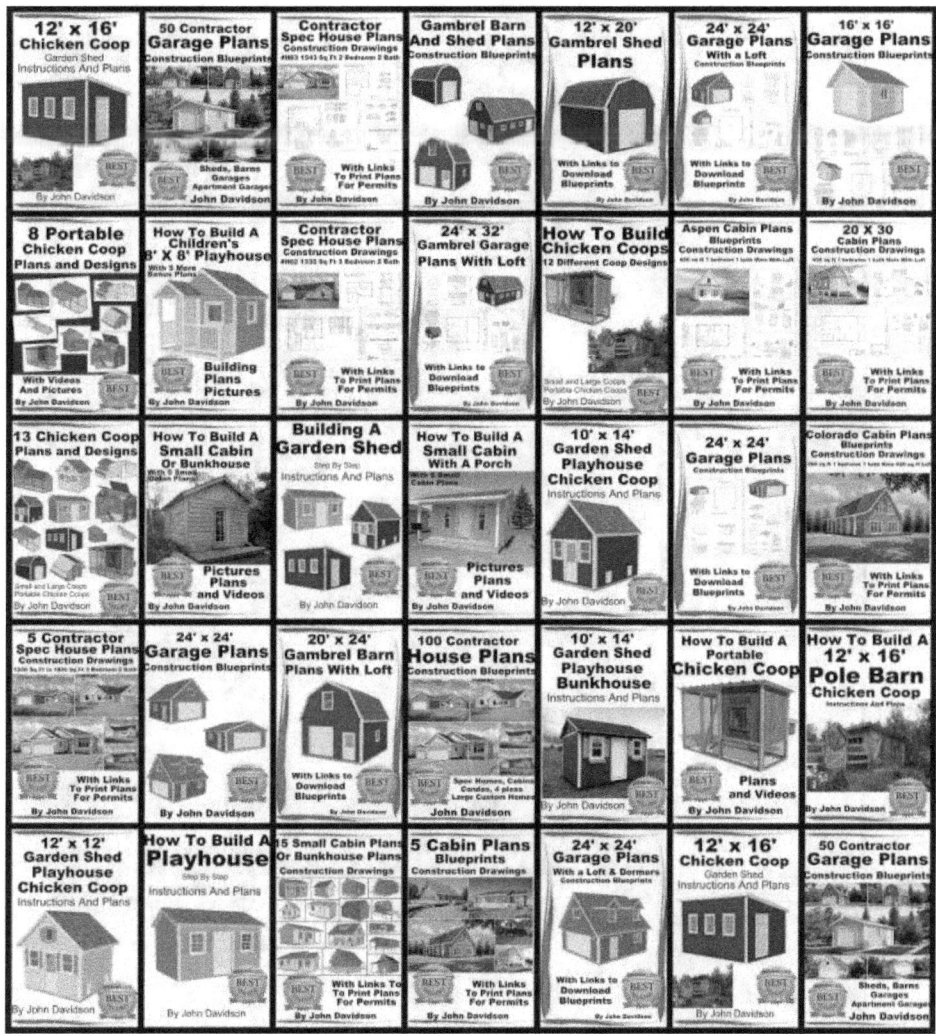

Entrepreneur Book Series

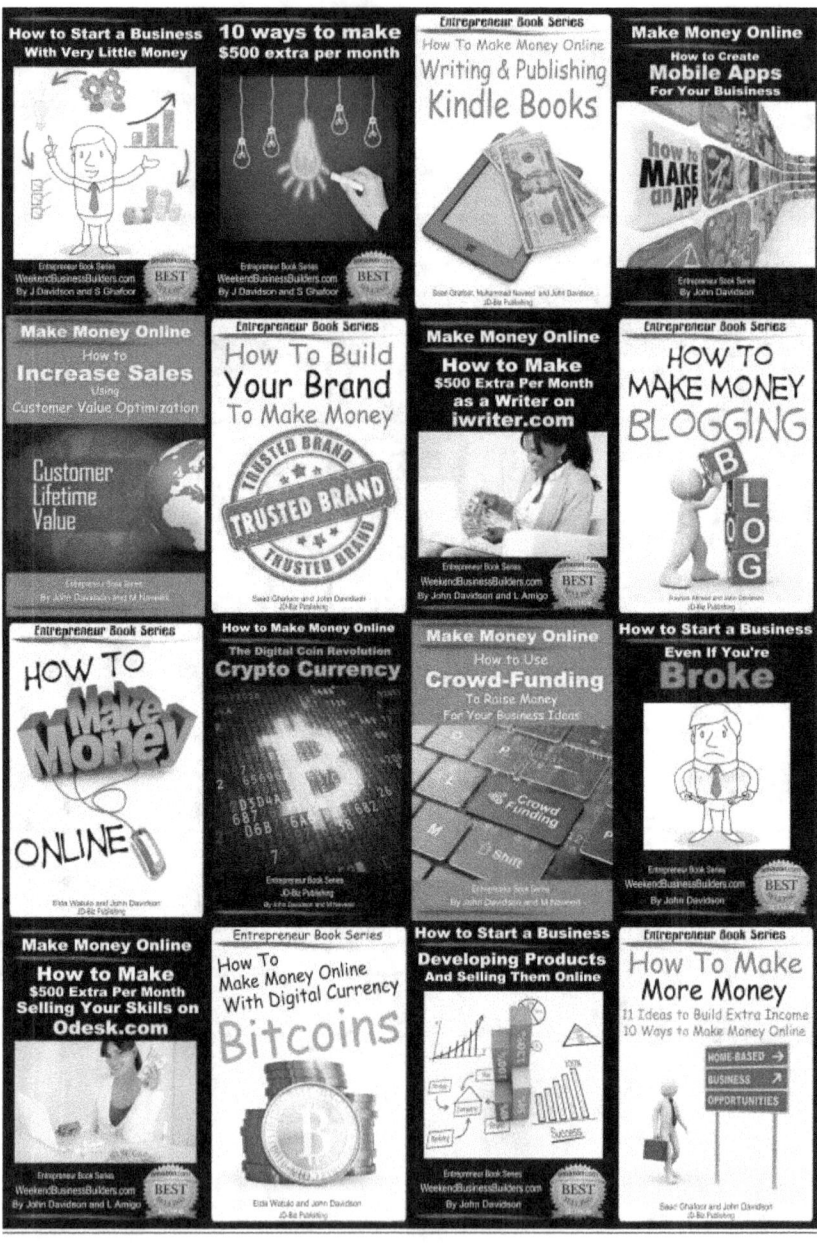

Our books are available at

1. Amazon.com

2. Barnes and Noble

3. Itunes

4. Kobo

5. Smashwords

6. Google Play Books

Publisher

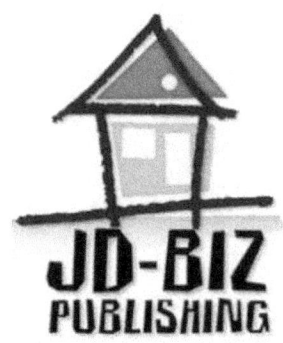

JD-Biz Corp

P O Box 374

Mendon, Utah 84325

http://www.jd-biz.com/

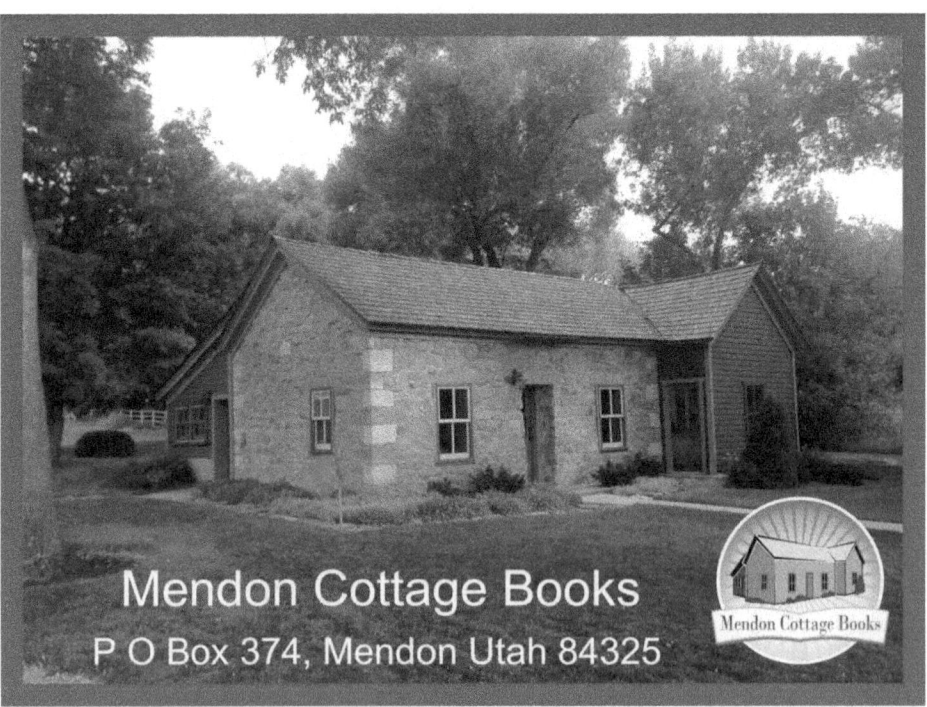

www.ingramcontent.com/pod-product-compliance
Lightning Source LLC
Chambersburg PA
CBHW070623290526
45790CB00002B/968